Rapid Midwifery

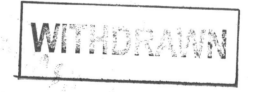

Rapid Midwifery

Sarah Snow
Principal Lecturer and Lead Midwife for Education
Oxford Brookes University

Kate Taylor
Senior Lecturer
University of Worcester

Jane Carpenter
Third year MSc pre-registration midwifery student
Oxford Brookes University

WILEY Blackwell

This edition first published 2016 © 2016 by John Wiley & Sons, Ltd

Registered office: John Wiley & Sons, Ltd, The Atrium, Southern Gate, Chichester, West Sussex, PO19 8SQ, UK

Editorial offices: 9600 Garsington Road, Oxford, OX4 2DQ, UK
The Atrium, Southern Gate, Chichester, West Sussex, PO19 8SQ, UK
111 River Street, Hoboken, NJ 07030-5774, USA

For details of our global editorial offices, for customer services and for information about how to apply for permission to reuse the copyright material in this book please see our website at www.wiley.com/wiley-blackwell

Library of Congress Cataloging-in-Publication Data

Names: Snow, Sarah, 1966- , author. | Taylor, Kate, 1951- , author. |
Carpenter, Jane, 1971- , author.
Title: Rapid midwifery / Sarah Snow, Kate Taylor, Jane Carpenter.
Description: Chichester, West Sussex, UK ; Hoboken, NJ : John Wiley & Sons
Inc., 2016. | Includes bibliographical references and index.
Identifiers: LCCN 2015047745| ISBN 9781119023364 (pbk.) | ISBN 9781119023371
(Adobe PDF) | ISBN 9781119023388 (epub)
Subjects: | MESH: Midwifery–methods | Handbooks
Classification: LCC RG950 | NLM WQ 165 | DDC 618.2–dc23 LC record available
at http://lccn.loc.gov/2015047745

9781119023364 [paperback]

A catalogue record for this book is available from the British Library.

Wiley also publishes its books in a variety of electronic formats. Some content that appears in print may not be available in electronic books.

Cover image: © Science Photo Library/Gettyimages

Set in 7.5/9.5pt, FrutigerLTStd-Light by SPi Global, Chennai, India
Printed and bound in Malaysia by Vivar Printing Sdn Bhd

1 2016

Contents

IV Hot Topics, 99

Conclusion: Top Tips for Examination Success, 115

Index, 119

Preface

Rapid Midwifery is part of a series of revision guides that has the fundamental aim of supporting student learning. This book is primarily aimed at pre-registration and post-experience midwifery students who are in the first or second year of their programme. Both years are challenging, especially when the realities of a midwifery course become apparent and students are adapting to the inherent professional, academic and social demands of their programme. During the first year, the relentless approach of the first assessment can instil great stress in students and may be a pivotal decision point in their continuing forwards on the programme. This book is aimed at alleviating some of that stress. By offering bite-sized information that is thoroughly supported by current best evidence, this book will be a helpful revision tool in preparing for looming OSCEs and written examinations.

Rapid Midwifery has two distinct features. First, it is written in sections that closely mimic assessment criteria used in midwifery examinations. Although each university sets its own criteria, examinations are set to test broadly a student's knowledge of key physiology; principles of safe and effective midwifery care; relevant underpinning evidence and professional accountability. Second, each topic has been mapped against the 6Cs, using *care* as the base point. Although each aspect of midwifery that is addressed within this book can be mapped against a number of the 6Cs, we have decided to identify what we consider to be the most predominant and therefore most relevant 'C'. We hope that this map will stimulate the reader to consider further their practice within the framework of compassionate midwifery care.

Rapid Midwifery is not a textbook, nor is it a complete and definitive guide to midwifery. It should be used wisely and strategically, alongside a wide range of other sources that explore the topics in greater breadth and depth. *Rapid Midwifery* is not designed to do anything more than support new midwifery students' revision and serve as an appetiser for the main course that is lifelong learning.

Sarah Snow
August 2015

Acknowledgement

We would like to extend our grateful thanks to Dr Martin Spurin, Programme Manager for the Youth, Community and Families degree programmes at University College Birmingham, who contributed the Conclusion to this book.

Midwifery Care

Compassion	Communication	Committment	Courage	Competence
Infections in pregnancy Minor disorders of pregnancy Promoting normality Contraception and sexual health Domestic abuse	Bio-physical tests Gestational diabetes First stage of labour Cord prolapse Postpartum haemorrhage Postnatal mental illness Obesity Sepsis	Pre-conceptual health Pharmacological and non-pharmacological analgesia Promoting normality	Anxiety and depression Shoulder dystocia Breech birth	Bleeding in pregnancy Intrahepatic cholestasis of pregnancy Pre-eclampsia Occipito-posterior position Second stage of labour Perineal trauma assessment Waterbirth Third stage of labour Recognising the deteriorating woman

Rapid midwifery compassionate care map – linked throughout the book with green highlighted text and adapted from the 6Cs: DH (2012) *Compassion in Practice*, Department of Health, London.

PART I

Antenatal Care

Rapid Midwifery, First Edition. Sarah Snow, Kate Taylor, and Jane Carpenter.
© 2016 John Wiley & Sons, Ltd. Published 2016 by John Wiley & Sons, Ltd.

Antenatal Health Assessment

The main objective of antenatal care is to support the woman through pregnancy and to monitor the health and well-being of the woman and fetus. Although pre-conceptual care is advised (see Section 1.10), antenatal care generally commences at booking. The National Institute for Health and Care Excellence (NICE) provides a framework and recommended schedules for routine antenatal care (NICE 2014c); however, timely referral is required if the woman or fetus is at increased risk. All care should be evidence based and woman centred, enabling her to make informed choices about her care.

KEY POINTS

- The first antenatal contact with the woman requires comprehensive history taking, including relevant obstetric, medical and personal details. Determining risk, offering an early ultrasound scan for gestational age, together with health screening checks and tests should be discussed (NICE 2014b).

- Blood pressure monitoring, urinalysis and abdominal examination are all essential components of antenatal care; however, other physical and emotional issues need to be considered.

- **Breast examination:** This is not routinely recommended (NICE 2014b); however, the woman may find information about breast changes to be reassuring. Breast tenderness and tingling often occur early in pregnancy and an early increase in size often occurs. Colostrum leakage is common.

- **Blood pressure:** A number of factors can influence blood pressure measurements, including time of day, size of cuff, maternal position and variations in technique. Midwives must fully understand the principal mechanisms that control blood pressure and other factors that can influence systolic and diastolic pressures, blood pressure phases and Korotkoff sounds.

- **Urinalysis:** Observation of the volume, colour, smell, deposits and specific gravity of urine offers a unique insight into the physiological workings of many body systems (Blows 2012).
  - **Colour:** This is dependent on concentration and varies from pale straw (normal) to amber. Diet, drugs, bilirubinuria and haematuria affect the colour of urine. Haematuria is not normal and may be indicative of infection or trauma.
  - **Clarity:** Urine should be clear. Cloudy or foamy urine can be caused by protein; cloudy and thick urine may be indicative of the presence of bacteria (Blows 2012). Routine midstream urine (MSU) screening for asymptomatic bacteriuria early in pregnancy to exclude asymptomatic pyelonephritis is currently recommended by NICE (2014b).
  - **Odour:** The odour of urine can be influenced by food. However, a smell of pear-drops or nail-polish remover indicates the presence of ketones which may be due to fasting, vomiting or uncontrolled diabetes mellitus. Infection may cause the urine to smell offensive and, when accompanied by the presence of nitrates and/or leucocytes on test strips, further laboratory culture is required.
  - **Specific gravity** is affected by both the water concentration and solute concentration in a urine sample and reflects the kidney's ability to concentrate or dilute urine.
  - **pH** reflects the acidity or alkalinity of urine and a low pH may predispose to the formation of calculi (stones) in the kidneys or bladder (Waugh and Grant 2014).

- Altered renal tubular function can increase renal excretion of glucose and protein. This needs to be considered when analysing urine.

- **Abdominal examination** is carried out from 24 weeks and is achieved by inspection, palpation and auscultation.
  - **Inspection:** The uterus should be ovoid in shape, being longer than it is broad. The size and shape of the abdomen can give clues to the size and position of the

fetus as pregnancy progresses. However, a full bladder, distended colon and obesity can make the assessment of fetal size difficult. Skin changes, such as linea nigra and striae gravidarum and scars from previous surgery, self-harm or domestic violence may be evident on abdominal inspection. Fetal movements may be reported from around 20 weeks (Bharj and Henshaw 2011).

o **Fundal palpation** determines the presence of a head or breech in the fundus. The head is hard and round and much more distinctive in outline than the breech.

o Symphysis–fundal height (SFH) should be measured (in centimetres) and recorded at each antenatal appointment from 24 weeks (NICE 2014b). Measurements should be plotted on a customised chart. Further investigation is required if a single measurement plots below the 10th centile or serial measurements show slow growth by crossing centiles (RCOG 2013).

o **Lateral palpation** determines the position of the fetal back. This feels like a smooth continuous line of resistance, while fetal limbs feel like small irregular shapes on the opposite side. The fetal back cannot be felt if the fetus is in the occipito-posterior position (see Section 2.1.2), although fetal limbs can be felt on both sides of the midline (Bharj and Henshaw 2011).

o **Pelvic palpation** determines the presentation of the fetus, the attitude and degree of engagement. This is best carried out using a two-hand approach. If the head is above the pelvic brim then the head is not engaged. Once engaged, if the fingers of one hand slide further into the pelvis than the other, then the head is flexed. NICE (2014b) recommends that presentation should not be assessed by abdominal palpation prior to 36 weeks.

• **Auscultation** of the fetal heart is best heard at a point over the fetal shoulder, hence lateral palpation to identify the fetal back is useful. When the fetus is in the occipito-posterior position, the fetal heart can be heard at the midline or lateral borders. NICE (2014b) does not recommend antenatal auscultation or electronic fetal heart rate monitoring in women with uncomplicated pregnancies.

• **Vaginal discharge** often increases in pregnancy. It is usually white, non-offensive and non-irritant. If the discharge is associated with pain on micturition, soreness, itching or an offensive smell, then further investigations are required (see Section 1.7).

• **Oedema** should not be present at the initial assessment. However, it may occur as pregnancy progresses due to physiological changes. Oedema that is visible in the woman's face and hands and becomes increasingly pitted in the lower limbs may be indicative of hypertension, especially if other markers are present.

• **Varicosities** are common in pregnancy owing to the effect of progesterone on the smooth muscles of blood vessel walls. Redness and tenderness/pain and areas that appear white may be indicative of deep vein thrombosis and require medical referral.

• **Maternal weight and height** should be measured at the first contact with the pregnant woman. Routine weighing during pregnancy is not recommended unless clinical management can be influenced or if nutrition is a concern (NICE 2014b). Women who have a body mass index (BMI) of <18 or ≥30 kg/m^2 need referral to a consultant and other health professionals working in nutrition and weight management (NICE 2010) (see Section 4.3).

ESSENTIALS OF MIDWIFERY CARE NICE (2014b) offers comprehensive guidance for the provision of antenatal care, a summary of which is provided below to aid revision.

• Management of care will depend on the individual needs of the woman. A holistic woman-centred approach is paramount and observations of physical characteristics are important, as these may give clues to current problems or problems that may arise.

- When women are assessed and remain low risk, a midwifery-led model of care should be offered.
- If problems arise, a clear referral pathway should be established to ensure that the woman is managed and treated by appropriate specialist team members (NICE 2014c).
- Urinalysis for protein should be carried out at each antenatal visit to screen for pre-eclampsia; however, routine urinalysis for glycosuria is not recommended as pregnancy affects glomerular filtration and exceeds the renal threshold for glucose (Blackburn 2013).
- Urinalysis is an everyday task in midwifery practice; however, its relevance in identifying underlying disease processes and infection should not be undervalued.
- Although formal fetal movement counting is not recommended, women should be encouraged to be aware of their baby's usual pattern of movements. The Royal College of Obstetricians and Gynaecologists (RCOG) gives guidance on the management of women with reduced fetal movements (RCOG 2011c).
- Ultrasound estimation for suspected large for gestational age babies is not recommended for low-risk women. However, the RCOG (2013) recommends that women with a single SFH that plots below the 10th centile or serial measurements that demonstrate slow or static growth by crossing centiles should be referred for ultrasound measurement of fetal size.
- Vaginal discharge should be differentiated from unexplained vaginal wetness to exclude amniotic fluid leak.

PROFESSIONAL ACCOUNTABILITY
- The midwife is required to facilitate and respect maternal choice. This can occur only if information is timely and appropriate.
- Midwives should be aware of local protocols and national guidelines to ensure that referral to appropriate members of the multidisciplinary team is made when deviations from the norm are identified.
- Accurate, contemporaneous documentation should reflect all care given and planned.

Further Resources

Geeky Medics. *How to Take an Accurate Blood Pressure*, https://www.youtube.com/watch?v=f6HtqolhKqo.

Anxiety and Depression

It is important to recognise that depression, anxiety and stress during pregnancy are at least as common as an altered emotional state during the puerperium. Glover (2014) identified that the emotional health of women during pregnancy remains a neglected aspect of maternity care. In addition, Brockington (1998) observed that the focus on the concept of 'postnatal depression' has detracted from the need to recognise and manage it like any other depressive illness that occurs during a woman's life span.

KEY POINTS

- Around 3–17% of women experience depressive illness during pregnancy (Leight *et al.* 2010).

- Mindfulness-based cognitive therapy is associated with a significant reduction in both the incidence and reoccurrence of depression. It may also be an effective strategy for women who do not respond to other therapies such as cognitive behavioural therapy (CBT) (Segal *et al.* 2012).

- Consideration and understanding of the context of a pregnant woman's anxiety or depression are crucial when determining care (Dunkel Schetter and Tanner 2012).

- Anxiety and depressive symptoms in pregnancy are associated with preterm birth and low birth weight infants (Dunkel Schetter and Tanner 2012).

- Evidence suggests that if a woman is stressed, anxious or depressed during pregnancy, her child is more likely to experience adverse outcomes, including emotional problems (O'Connor *et al.* 2002) and cognitive impairment (van den Bergh and Marcoen 2004).

- The Family Nurse Partnership (2015) remains the only intervention that starts in pregnancy and is associated with improved outcomes for child behaviour (Glover 2014). It also has one of the most robust evidence bases for successful interventions with the care of vulnerable parents and babies.

- The Mind 'Building Resilience for Better Mental Health' project reports that supporting pregnant women and new mothers to adopt strategies that manage altered mood helps them to stay well (Steen *et al.* 2015).

ESSENTIALS OF MIDWIFERY CARE

- NICE (2014a) offers a number of recommendations for the care and support of women, including:

  ○ Asking questions that are designed to identify depression as part of the general discussion about the woman's mental health at booking. This may then trigger referral to her GP or mental health professional. Examples of such questions include: *During the past month, have you often been bothered by feeling down, depressed or hopeless? During the past month, have you often been bothered by having little interest or pleasure in doing things?*

  ○ Providing information to the woman and her partner about mental health during pregnancy, including treatment and prevention options, for example, psychological interventions and medication.

  ○ Monitoring symptoms regularly throughout pregnancy and referring women where appropriate for facilitated, self-help interventions. More severe symptoms may require high-intensity psychological interventions such as CBT.

  ○ Involving the woman (and her partner/family) in all aspects of her care and acknowledging the woman's central role in decision-making.

  ○ Recognising the impact of any mental health issue on the woman's relationship with her partner and family.

○ Developing an integrated care plan that clearly sets out the care and treatment of the mental health problem. This includes the involvement of other agencies, for example, mental health services.

PROFESSIONAL ACCOUNTABILITY

- Asking pregnant women sensitive questions about their mental health requires courage; however, a midwife's duty of care encompasses all aspects of a woman's mental and physical health.

- Record keeping is an important aspect of caring for women with mental health needs and these records may not be conventional written ones. For example, women may value a record of their consultation in a variety of formats, e.g. audio, visual or verbal (NICE 2014a).

- When working with girls and young women who disclose mental health issues, midwives must be clear about local and national guidelines regarding confidentiality and safeguarding.

Further Resources

Family Nurse Partnership,
    http://fnp.nhs.uk/.

Bio-physical Tests
Blood Tests

Blood tests in pregnancy fall into two main categories, diagnostic and screening. NICE (2014b) further categorises blood testing into screening for haematological conditions, screening for haemoglobinopathies, screening for Down syndrome (and other trisomies) and screening for infection. Some blood tests are routinely offered at the initial assessment. Others are offered at specific times during pregnancy or as indicated, in order to determine and manage the sequelae of specific complications. At the initial antenatal assessment, women are also routinely offered screening for certain infections (see Section 1.10).

Blood tests offered at the initial assessment include the following.

ABO Blood Group and Rhesus (Rh) Factor

KEY POINTS
- What determines a blood group is the presence or absence of a range of different proteins (antigens) on the red blood cell membrane.
- Antigens on the red blood cell membrane can stimulate an immune response from antibodies in the plasma if transferred from one individual to another (Waugh and Grant 2014), in this instance between mother to baby.
- Confirmation of a woman's blood group and Rh status is necessary to prevent a potentially fatal transfusion reaction (should a blood transfusion be required) and to prevent haemolytic disease of the newborn (HDN)[1] (Qureshi *et al.* 2014).
- Determined by genetic control, the Rh grouping system involves many different antigens (which produce antibodies), with D being the most potent antigen and the one most commonly involved in incompatibility between mother and fetus causing HDN.

ESSENTIALS OF MIDWIFERY CARE Both the British Committee for Standards in Haematology (Qureshi *et al.* 2014) and the RCOG (2014) give guidance for the management of women with red cell antibodies during pregnancy. It is essential that midwives are aware of the following in order to provide effective care:

- To reduce the incidence of HDN, women should be screened for atypical red cell alloantibodies early in pregnancy and again at 28 weeks, regardless of RhD status.
- All RhD-negative women should be offered antenatal anti-D immunoglobulin (Ig) prophylaxis in accordance with local guidelines for dosage and timing of administration (NICE 2014b). If a sensitising episode should occur, for example, miscarriage, amniocentesis or external cephalic version, further administration of anti-D is required and within 72 hours of the event (Qureshi *et al.* 2014; RCOG 2014).
- The amount of anti-D required is assessed by a Kleihauer blood test, which confirms the presence and estimates the number of fetal cells in the maternal circulation.
- Consideration should be given to offering testing to the woman's partner in order to determine whether anti-D prophylaxis is necessary (NICE 2014b), although this can be a sensitive paternity issue.

Full Blood Count

KEY POINTS
- A full blood count is one of the most common blood tests taken in pregnancy as it can provide important 'clues' to a woman's general health.

---

[1] Haemolytic disease of the newborn is an immune-mediated breakdown of red blood cells that occurs in Rhesus and ABO incompatibility.

- There are three types of blood cells: erythrocytes (red cells and the most abundant), platelets (thrombocytes) and leucocytes (white cells).
- Haemoglobin (Hb) is the most frequently referred to index (Blann 2006), with almost the entire weight of an erythrocyte (red blood cell) consisting of haemoglobin.
- Each haemoglobin molecule consists of a pigmented iron-containing complex called haem and a polypeptide protein (globulin). The iron atoms play a key role in the oxygen-carrying capacity of erythrocytes (Waugh and Grant 2014).
- Physiological anaemia describes a fall in Hb concentration due to the physiological changes that occur in normal pregnancy.
- If the concentration of erythrocytes is low, as indicated by the red cell count (RCC), this may also be indicative of anaemia. If concentrations are high, then polycythaemia should be considered.
- When the mean cell volume (MCV) is low, then serum ferritin levels should be investigated. Serum ferritin is a stable glycoprotein that accurately reflects iron stores.
- Iron deficiency represents a spectrum of anaemias ranging from iron depletion to iron deficiency anaemia (Pavord et al. 2012).
- Abnormal clinical findings may indicate a spectrum of anaemic disorders, polycythaemia or congenital haemoglobinopathies such as sickle cell disease and thalassaemia (Blann 2006).
- Leucocytes are normally found in low concentrations; however, rising white cell numbers usually indicate infection or trauma. They therefore play an important role in the body's defence mechanism.
- Other white blood cells include neutrophils, which protect the body from bacterial invasion; eosinophils, which have a specialist role in the elimination of parasites; basophils, which are associated with allergic reactions; and monocytes, which defend the body from bacterial, fungal and other pathogens by phagocytosis.
- Lymphocytes make immunoglobulins (antibodies capable of recognising and attacking invading pathogens) and aid antibody production (Blann 2006).
- Platelets (thrombocytes) play an important role in haemostasis. Platelets quickly adhere to each other when blood vessels are damaged, releasing substances that attract more platelets to the site to form a platelet plug (Waugh and Grant 2014).

ESSENTIALS OF MIDWIFERY CARE

- A full blood count is taken at the initial assessment and routinely during pregnancy, typically at 28 weeks (NICE 2014b).
- NICE (2014b) recommends that when Hb levels fall outside the normal range for pregnancy (11 g/100 ml at first contact and 10.5 g/100 ml at 28 weeks), this should be investigated and iron supplementation considered.
- Routine iron supplementation for all women is not recommended in the United Kingdom. However, all women should be given dietary information to maximise iron intake and absorption (Pavord et al. 2012).
- In pregnancy, platelet levels may fall but usually remain within the normal range for non-pregnant women. A rise may be indicative of infection and an abnormal decrease should be viewed with suspicion and therefore investigated (Boyle 2011).

Haemoglobinopathies are a complex group of genetically acquired conditions. They occur in individuals who inherit two haemoglobin gene variants which lead to the synthesis of abnormal haemoglobin and increased red cell membrane fragility. The resulting reductions in the oxygen-carrying capacity and life span of the red cells are characteristics of sickle cell anaemia and thalassaemia (Blackburn 2013).

Sickle Cell Disease

KEY POINTS

- Sickle cell disease (SCD) exhibits geographical variations, with the highest prevalence amongst those of Black African and Black Caribbean family origin. Sickle cell disease affects 1 in every 2000 births in England (NHS 2011).
- The pattern of inheritance is such that one gene from each parent (homozygous genotype for HbSS) results in a sickle cell-positive offspring.
- Offspring who inherit one gene (heterozygote) have sickle cell trait (HbAS) and usually do not display the disease (Yerby 2010a).
- In SCD, the characteristic sickle-shaped erythrocytes result when abnormal, deoxygenated haemoglobin molecules become misshaped.
- Sickle cells do not move smoothly through the circulation and therefore cause an obstruction to blood flow, resulting in intravascular clotting, tissue ischaemia and infarction (Waugh and Grant 2014).
- Normal haematological, cardiovascular, renal and respiratory changes during pregnancy place the woman and infant at greater risk of 'sickle crises' and complications such as an increased risk of thromboembolic events, antepartum haemorrhage and pre-eclampsia.
- Fetal and neonatal complications such as prematurity and growth restriction may arise due to placental infarction and fetal hypoxia (RCOG 2011a; Blackburn 2013).

Thalassaemias

KEY POINTS

- Thalassaemias are a group of hereditary haemolytic anaemias, most prevalent in those of Mediterranean, African-Caribbean, Chinese and Asian origin.
- They are characterised by an impaired and unbalanced synthesis of either the two α-globin or two β-globin chains (Waugh and Grant 2014).
- The phenotype and severity of those with α-thalassaemia are dependent on the number of missing or altered genes involved in α-chain production.
- Those with one or two affected genes have either a silent presentation or mild anaemia. If all four genes are missing, the fetus cannot synthesise either normal fetal haemoglobin or adult haemoglobin. These infants develop cardiac failure and hydrops fetalis and are often stillborn.
- Until stem cell transplants are readily available, affected individuals require lifelong blood transfusions (Blackburn 2013).
- β-Thalassaemia major results from the inheritance of a defective β-globin gene from each parent and therefore the fetus is homozygous.
- This results in a severe transfusion-dependent anaemia. Many girls with thalassaemia major die in childhood or adolescence and those who survive are often amenorrheic and infertile.
- The heterozygous state, β-thalassaemia trait (thalassaemia minor) causes mild to moderate microcytic anaemia. Those affected are generally asymptomatic, although haemoglobin levels are reduced.

ESSENTIALS OF MIDWIFERY CARE Both sickle cell and β-thalassaemia major can restrict a child's or adult's ability to conduct normal daily activities. The NHS sickle cell and thalassaemia screening programme (NHS 2011) sets out standards for antenatal and newborn screening and the RCOG (2011a) guideline makes recommendations for the management of sickle cell disease in pregnancy. These, together with the RCOG (2014) *Management of Beta Thalassaemia in Pregnancy* provide evidence-based guidance for care:

- Information about screening for sickle cell diseases and thalassaemias, including the implications of carrier status, should be given to pregnant women at the first contact with the midwife, ideally before 10 weeks.

- In low-prevalence trusts, a family origin questionnaire (FOQ) should be used to assess risk. In high-prevalence trusts, all pregnant women should also be offered screening.

- When the woman is identified as being affected or a carrier, the father of the baby should also be offered screening.

- Care for all women whose pregnancy is complicated by any form of haemoglobinopathy should be provided by a multidisciplinary team including an obstetrician, a midwife with experience of high-risk antenatal care and a haematologist with an interest in haemoglobinopathies (RCOG 2011a, 2014).

Screening tests for Down (T21), Edwards (T18) and Patau (T13) Syndromes

KEY POINTS

- Where a fault during meiosis occurs, three copies of a chromosome may result and give rise to a named trisomy (Waugh and Grant 2014), for example, Down syndrome. In the United Kingdom, all pregnant women are therefore offered antenatal screening.

- The eligibility criterion for Down syndrome screening is all women with a singleton or twin pregnancy at ≤20+0 weeks. The eligibility criterion for Edwards and Patau syndromes is all women with singleton or twin pregnancy at <14+1 weeks. In each case, the gestational age in weeks must be confirmed by ultrasound scan (Public Health England 2015).

- Women presenting in the first trimester between 10+0 and 14+1 weeks are offered the combined test to calculate the risk of the pregnancy being affected by Down, Edwards and Patau syndromes.

- The combined test uses maternal age, the nuchal translucency (NT) measurement and two biochemical markers, together with gestational age, which is calculated from the fetal crown–rump length (CRL).

- Women presenting between 14+2 and 20+0 weeks are offered the quadruple test for Down (T21) syndrome only. The optimal time for this test is 16 weeks.

- The quadruple test uses maternal age and four biochemical markers, including AFP and hCG.

ESSENTIALS OF MIDWIFERY CARE Both NICE (2014b) and the NHS fetal anomaly screening programme (FASP) offer guidance regarding anomaly screening (Public Health England 2015). A summary of this guidance is provided below.

- Women should be given information about screening at the first contact with the midwife and understand that the choice to embark on screening remains with them.

- Women should be informed that screening does not provide a definitive diagnosis and an explanation regarding risk scoring should be given. Nationally agreed screening protocols use a cut-off of 1:150 at term.

- In cases where screening is accepted, but it is not possible to obtain the NT measurement at the first attempt, at least one other attempt should be offered.

- The midwife should be aware of varying screening pathways, the NHS FASP and their local trust arrangements. For example, for first trimester tests, maternal blood may be taken (within the recommended parameters) prior to the ultrasound scan or the blood test can be taken at the same time as the ultrasound scan. The laboratory takes prime responsibility for the risk calculation.

- When results are low risk, women should be notified within 2 weeks of the test being taken.
- When results are high risk, the woman should be notified within 3 days and offered face-to-face discussion with a suitably experienced health professional to discuss her care options. Prompt referral should be made to an obstetrician with specialist knowledge in fetal medicine.
- Women with a high-risk result should be offered diagnostic testing which they can decline or accept. This should be documented. Good clinical practice is to obtain formal written consent for the procedure.
  - Chorionic villus sampling (CVS) and amniocentesis are both invasive diagnostic procedures performed under continuous ultrasound guidance.
  - CVS can be carried out between 10 and 15 weeks and amniocentesis is usually performed after 15 weeks of pregnancy.
  - Both carry risk of miscarriage and the woman must be made fully aware of the relative risks of undertaking either of these invasive procedures.
- The woman must be informed that diagnostic testing will give results for Down, Edwards and Patau syndromes irrespective of the initial screening choices.

Ultrasound

KEY POINTS
- All pregnant women should be offered an early ultrasound scan between 10+0 and 13+6 weeks to determine gestation and to detect multiple pregnancies.
- Crown–rump length (CRL) measurements should be used to determine gestational age. If the CRL is more than 84 mm, the gestational age should be determined using head circumference.
- The CRL can influence the timing of nuchal translucency measurements. A CRL measurement of less than 45.0 mm requires recall for a further scan. If the CRL is greater than 84.0 mm, second trimester anomaly tests should be offered.
- The NHS FASP recommends that a mid-pregnancy scan should be offered between 18+0 and 20+6 weeks of pregnancy to screen for major fetal anomalies (Public Health England 2015).
- The main structures that are assessed can indicate a number of specific conditions and women may choose to be screened for all or only some of these.

ESSENTIALS OF MIDWIFERY CARE Both NICE (2014b) and the NHS FASP (Public Health England 2015) offer guidance regarding anomaly screening, summarised below to aid revision:
- Midwives should inform women of the conditions that can be screened for.
- Women should be informed of the limitations of routine ultrasound screening and that detection rates vary by the type of fetal anomaly, the woman's BMI and the position of the unborn baby at the time of scan.
- Some fetal anomalies will be confirmed by scan alone, others will require prenatal, invasive, diagnostic testing.
- When routine ultrasound screening is performed to detect neural tube defects, α-fetoprotein testing is not required.

- If fetal anomaly is suspected or detected, the woman should be informed at the time of the scan by either the sonographer or the midwife to discuss further investigations.
- The discussion should include sufficient information to ensure that the woman is aware of the purpose, benefits, limitations and implications of undergoing further investigations.
- The woman should be referred to an obstetrician with an interest in fetal medicine within 3 days or should be referred to a tertiary unit by the obstetrician within 5 days.
- Women should be counselled and supported in their decision to terminate or continue the pregnancy. Referral to appropriate paediatric and support services should be made.

Other Biophysical Tests

A number of tests can be carried out during the antenatal period to assess fetal well-being. Tests may include fetal movement monitoring, fetal heart rate activity, growth scans, Doppler ultrasound and assessment of amniotic fluid volume. Although these tests are not routinely performed, one or a combination can be utilised when there are concerns in order to optimise care and the time of birth.

KEY POINTS

- **A biophysical profile (BPP)** uses ultrasound to assess five variables: fetal movement; tone; breathing; the amniotic fluid volume; and heart rate activity.
- Each variable is assigned a maximum score of 2. A total score between 8 and 10 indicates a potentially healthy fetus; a score of 6 or less is suspicious (Lalor *et al.* 2008).
- A BPP is used to aid detection of central nervous system depression in the fetus.
- A modified profile (MBPP) may be used first; this involves a CTG to monitor heart rate activity, plus assessment of amniotic fluid volume.
- **Fetal movements** are a sign of fetal well-being. Most women are aware of fetal movements by 20 weeks' gestation (multiparous women usually by 16 weeks and primiparous by 20 weeks) (RCOG 2011c).
- Fetal movements can be defined as discrete kicks, flutters, a swish or a roll. Changes in the number and nature of fetal movements as the fetus matures are a reflection of normal neurological development (Blackburn 2013).
- **Fetal heart rate activity** can be an indication of fetal well-being if certain parameters are met. Features of a reassuring fetal heart rate include a baseline rate between 100 and 160 beats per minute; baseline variability of 5 or more; accelerations and no decelerations (NICE 2014b).
- **Growth scans:** Diagnosis of a small for gestational age fetus usually relies on ultrasound measurement of fetal abdominal circumference (AC) or estimation of fetal weight (EFW). Where the fetal AC or EFW is <10th centile or there is evidence of reduced growth velocity, women should be offered serial assessment of fetal size and umbilical artery Doppler (RCOG 2013).
- **Doppler ultrasound** provides a non-invasive insight into feto-maternal circulation. Normally, the umbilical artery presents low resistance to blood flow and this is indicated by a low PI (pulsatile index) and therefore a desirable high profusion. A high PI indicates increased resistance and low profusion (Stampalija *et al.* 2010).
- **Amniotic fluid volume** is estimated by measuring the single vertical pocket. Alternatively, an amniotic fluid index (AFI) can be estimated by measuring the liquor in each of four quadrants around the fetus which are devoid of umbilical cord or fetal parts. An AFI of <5–6 cm is defined as oligohydramnious and is associated with growth restriction, some congenital anomalies and post-maturity. An AFI of >24 cm is defined as polyhydramnios and is associated with some congenital anomalies, maternal diabetes, multiple pregnancies and hydrops fetalis (Blackburn 2013).

ESSENTIALS OF MIDWIFERY CARE The use of the biophysical profile test for high-risk pregnancies is controversial; however, there can be no doubt of the value of timely fetal surveillance. It is essential that midwives are able to recognise deviations from the norm, make sound clinical judgements and then institute timely referral to appropriate members of the multidisciplinary team.

- A biophysical profile is usually reserved for those pregnancies deemed high risk. However, there may be more than one reason for abnormal findings.
- Women should be advised of the need to be aware of fetal movements up to and including the onset of labour and to report any changes (RCOG 2011c).
- Accurate assessment of fetal heart rate is essential as this may affect a plan of care. NICE (2014b) does not support the use of routine, antenatal, electronic fetal heart rate monitoring for women with uncomplicated pregnancies.
- In high-risk pregnancies, a uterine artery Doppler ultrasound at 20–24 weeks of pregnancy has moderate predictive value for the severely small for gestational age neonate. Other indications for referral for Doppler ultrasound include oligohydramnious, disparity in fetal growth in multiple pregnancies, previous intrauterine growth restriction (IUGR) and some maternal conditions.
- A clinical assessment of amniotic fluid can be made during abdominal palpation in the second and third trimesters. Suspicion of either oligohydramnious or polyhydramnios needs referral for ultrasound evaluation.

ADDITIONAL EVIDENCE POINTS
- Non-invasive fetal genotyping using maternal blood is now possible for many blood cell antigens. This test should be performed in the first instance for the relevant antigen when maternal red cell antibodies are present (RCOG 2014).
- Sickle cell disease remains a high-risk condition. Chase *et al.* (2010) suggested that successful pregnancy outcomes can be achieved for women with SCD and that early access to specialist antenatal care is essential.
- Lalor *et al.* (2008) reviewed trials that compared BPP or MBPP with conventional monitoring (CTG) in outcomes of high- risk pregnancies. They were unable to come to any firm conclusion about the benefits or otherwise of BPP as a test of fetal well-being.

PROFESSIONAL ACCOUNTABILITY
- Midwives need to gain informed consent for all procedures.
- Midwives are required to make timely referral to appropriate members of the multidisciplinary team.
- Midwives need to be aware of national and local guidelines in order to deliver evidence-based care.
- Sensitive counselling and support should be given to the woman and her partner.
- The NMC Code (NMC 2015) requires midwives to document all care, identifying risk to ensure that colleagues who use the records have all the information they need. Therefore, communication is a vital requirement of effective care.

Further Resources

Down's Syndrome Association, http://www.downs-syndrome.org.uk/.

Sickle Cell Society, http://sicklecellsociety.org/.

United Kingdom Thalassaemia Society, http://ukts.org/home.html.

Bleeding in Pregnancy

Any degree of bleeding in pregnancy is not normal and needs urgent attention in order to identify and manage the cause. This cannot always be identified, however antenatal bleeding of unknown origin (ABUO) is by far the most common form of antepartum haemorrhage (Bhandari *et al.* 2014). Antepartum haemorrhage (APH) is defined as bleeding from or in the genital tract that occurs from 24 weeks' gestation and prior to the birth of the baby; placenta praevia and placental abruption are significant causes (RCOG 2011d). Bleeding before the 24th week of pregnancy can be caused by implantation, abortion, hydatidiform mole, cervical lesions, vaginitis and ectopic pregnancy (Hutcherson 2011).

Both RCOG guidelines cited in this section (RCOG 2011d, e) are supported by a comprehensive evidence base. Although both focus mainly on the two most important causes of bleeding in pregnancy, these are not the most common. As APH complicates 3–5% of pregnancies and is the leading cause of perinatal and maternal mortality worldwide, bleeding due to other causes is significant. Studies by McCormack *et al.* (2008) and Bhandari *et al.* (2014) that examined the consequences of antepartum bleeding of unknown origin are therefore also highly relevant.

KEY POINTS

- **Abruption** is more likely to be related to conditions that occur during pregnancy (Yang *et al.* 2009).
- Predisposing risk factors are numerous and include:
  - previous history of abruption;
  - bleeding in the first trimester;
  - pre-eclampsia;
  - fetal growth restriction;
  - non-vertex presentation;
  - polyhydramnios;
  - advanced maternal age;
  - premature rupture of membranes;
  - substance use (RCOG 2011e).
- When placental abruption occurs, a haematoma is formed that separates the placenta from the maternal vascular system. The bleeding can be revealed or concealed or a combination of both. Note that blood loss is often underestimated.
- The uterus will be hard and woody on palpation and may be tender, and the woman usually experiences pain. Blood loss is darker than that seen in placenta praevia (Yerby 2010c).
- **Placenta praevia** is implicated in one-third of all cases of APH and is more likely to be related to conditions that existed prior to pregnancy (Yang *et al.* 2009). It is a consequence of unusual development and implantation of the placenta, including vasa praevia[2] and velamentous cord insertion. Vasa praevia is associated with significant risk to the fetus. The loss of small amounts of blood can have a major impact on the fetus given that the fetal blood volume at term is around 80–100 ml/kg (Blackburn 2013).
- Risk factors include:
  - placental anomalies;
  - multiple pregnancy;
  - *in vitro* fertilisation (RCOG 2011e);

---

[2] Vasa praevia describes fetal vessels that run through the membrane unprotected by placental tissue or the umbilical cord.

- º previous caesarean section;
- º maternal age;
- º previous placenta praevia (Yerby 2010c).

- Placenta praevia is classified by the degree to which the placenta covers or partially covers the internal cervical os. If the placenta wholly covers the os then it is considered major praevia. If the leading edge of the placenta is in the lower uterine segment but not covering the os, it is classified as minor or partial praevia (RCOG 2011e).

- Marginal to major signs and symptoms of placenta praevia include: a painless, bright red blood loss, a non-tender or tense abdomen, fetal malpresentation and a non-engaged presenting part (RCOG 2011e).

- APH, particularly major haemorrhage in cases of abruption, can result in fetal hypoxia and abnormalities of the fetal heart pattern in addition to maternal collapse.

- Disseminated intravascular coagulation (DIC) is a significant concern when haemorrhage occurs.

- All women at risk of pre-term birth between 24 and 34+6 weeks should be given antenatal corticosteroids to reduce neonatal morbidity.

- A Kleihauer test should be taken in all cases when women are RhD negative in order to determine the dose of anti-D immunoglobulin required (see Section 1.3.1).

ESSENTIALS OF MIDWIFERY CARE Both of the RCOG Green-top Guidelines (RCOG 2011d,e) offer care management guidance for antepartum haemorrhage. A summary is provided below to aid revision:

- Women should be made aware of the importance of reporting any blood loss during pregnancy.

- Women need to be aware early in pregnancy that pregnancy can be unpredictable and, if haemorrhage is significant, a transfusion may be necessary.

- Anti-D should be given to all RhD-negative women in addition to any routine prophylactic doses already given.

- Women should be managed according to their individual needs.

- Midwives need to be aware of predisposing causes and risks associated with both placental abruption and placenta praevia.

- Women should be advised and encouraged to change modifiable risk factors such as smoking and drug use.

- Midwives need to be vigilant and aware that trauma may be a result of domestic violence (see Section 4.2).

- Haemoglobin levels below the normal UK range for pregnancy should be investigated and iron supplementation considered.

- Midwives need to be aware that young, fit, pregnant women with significant haemorrhage compensate remarkably well and therefore hypotension is always a very late sign of hypovolaemia (Paterson-Brown and Bamber 2014).

- A multidisciplinary team, including midwifery, obstetric, neonatal and anaesthetic staff, and haematology are required.

- When haemorrhage is significant, blood tests are required for full blood count (FBC) and coagulation screen, cross-match, urea and electrolytes and liver function tests (LFTs).

- Blood transfusion requirements should be based on full clinical assessment as initial haemoglobin levels may not reflect the amount of blood loss.

- Antenatal haemorrhage of unknown origin poses particular challenges; however, all women who present with bleeding in pregnancy should be referred for prompt consultant review.
- Placental location is usually identified at routine ultrasound scanning at 20 weeks. Definitive diagnosis of placenta praevia relies on follow-up imaging and this can influence the management of care.
- Vaginal and rectal examination should be avoided for women with placenta praevia and they should be advised against penetrative sexual intercourse.
- Blood loss can be defined as:
  - spotting;
  - minor, <50 ml that has settled;
  - major, 50–100 ml, with no signs of clinical shock;
  - massive, >1000 ml and/or signs of clinical shock.
- Clinical shock and the presence of fetal compromise or fetal demise are important indicators of volume depletion.
- The midwife must be aware of any signs or predisposing risk of DIC and be aware of the signs of coagulation failure (Hutcherson 2011).
- In cases of hypovolaemic shock, fluid replacement and correction of lost coagulation factors are essential (Ferns 2007).
- Emergency delivery may be indicated to aid resuscitation of the woman, as the gravid uterus limits venous return and cardiac output and also limits the effectiveness of cardiac compressions (Billington and Stevenson 2007).
- The fetal heart rate should be assessed once the woman is stable or resuscitation has commenced. The appropriate mode of delivery can then be determined.

PROFESSIONAL ACCOUNTABILITY
- Appropriate and prompt action and referral are essential in all cases of bleeding in pregnancy.
- Transfer to delivery suite rather than A&E is required for all women experiencing APH in the community. Delivery suite should be alerted in order to ensure that the appropriate multiprofessional team is in attendance.
- Midwives should be aware of current local and national guidelines for the management of obstetric haemorrhage and attend regular emergency skills drills to optimise timely and effective care.
- Documentation and communication are essential.
- Women, their families and the midwives caring for them may welcome debriefing.
- The NMC Code (NMC 2015) charges all nurses and midwives to work within their limits of competence … *to make timely and appropriate referral to another practitioner when it is in the best interest of the individual needing any action, care or treatment.*

Fetal Growth and Development

The potential for new life begins at fertilisation and culminates with the birth of the baby. This remarkable journey begins when two gametes unite and takes around 266 days (38 weeks), during which time the transformation from zygote to embryo is complex. The development from embryo to fetus takes almost 9 weeks and results in the formation of all the major body systems. External features become established and begin to develop and a recognisable human being can be seen on ultrasound scan.

Growth throughout the fetal period is rapid and there is further differentiation of body structures and a gradual increase in functionality by week 20. From 20 weeks to term, further maturation of organ body systems occurs. This growth and development are dependent on factors such as genetic determination, maternal health and nutrition, availability of growth substrates, hormones and vascular support via the placenta (Moore and Persaud 2003a; Blackburn 2013). Clinically, the gestational period of embryonic and fetal development is calculated from the first day of the last menstrual period, which equates to 280 days (40 weeks) and is divided into three trimesters.

KEY POINTS

- *Week 9*: The crown–rump length is approximately 5 cm. The head is large and measures half the fetal crown–rump length. External genitalia are not distinguishable and intestinal coils may still be outside the body cavity. The eyes are fused and the ears are low set.

- *Week 10*: Intestinal coils have all re-entered the body cavity. If this does not occur, the abdominal wall fails to close and the baby is born with exomphalos or gastroschisis.

- *Week 12*: The fetal length has more than doubled. The upper limbs have reached a length proportional to the fetal trunk; however, the lower limbs remain short. External genitalia begin to appear. Erythropoiesis decreases in the liver and now begins in the spleen. Formation and excretion of urine begin and the fetus swallows the amniotic fluid. Primary ossification centres of the skull and long bones develop and the beginning of fetal muscle movement occurs.

- *Weeks 13–16*: These are a period of rapid growth. The head is now proportionally smaller than the trunk and the lower limbs are nearing their correct proportions. There is active ossification of the skeleton and coordinated limb movements now occur. The eyes and ears are closer to normal positions and slow eye movements begin. External genitalia are now apparent and the differentiated ovaries contain primordial follicles.

- *Weeks 17–20*: Fetal growth slows. Limbs reach mature proportions and fetal movements are felt by the mother. The skin is covered in a protective layer of vernix caseosa. Lanugo covers the whole body by 20 weeks and hair and eyebrows are visible. Brown fat deposits are formed.

- *Weeks 21–25*: The fetus gains weight but the skin lacks subcutaneous fat and is therefore wrinkled, red and translucent. The fetus now has periods of sleep and activity. Rapid eye movement begins and blink–startle responses to sound occur. Surfactant secretions begin and although the respiratory system remains immature the fetus may still be viable if born prematurely. Fingernails are present.

- *Weeks 26–29*: The central nervous system can control breathing and intrauterine respiratory movements are made. The lungs are capable of breathing air, allowing gaseous exchange. Erythropoiesis moves from spleen to bone marrow. White subcutaneous fat is laid down under the skin. Head and lanugo hair is well established, eyes are open and toenails are visible.

- *Weeks 30–34*: White fat increases and now constitutes up to 8% of body weight. The skin is pink, opaque and smooth. Pupillary light reflex is present and lanugo disappears from the face. The fetus begins to store iron from 32 weeks. Most fetuses born at this gestation will survive.

- *Weeks 35–40*: The circumferences of the head and abdomen are approximately the same. By 38 weeks, body fat is about 16% of the body weight. The skin appears bluish pink and body lanugo disappears. Breast tissue is present in both sexes and, in the male, testes are in the scrotum. Nails reach the tips of the fingers and the fetus will have a firm grasp. (Moore and Persaud 2003a, b; Stables 2010; Coad and Dunstall 2012).

- Maternal conditions known to be associated with poor fetal growth and development include hypertension, chronic renal disease, diabetes, sickle cell anaemia, severe cardiac disease and malnutrition.

- Any condition that restricts placental perfusion and blood flow can have an adverse effect. When blood flow is poor, the blood is redirected to the brain at the expense of other tissue, resulting in asymmetric growth. This redistribution does not completely protect brain function so some abnormal neurological development may occur (Coad and Dunstall 2012).

- Other conditions that affect fetal growth and development include hyperthyroidism, hypothyroidism and phenylketonuria.

- Alcohol, smoking and drug misuse are all known to have adverse effects on the developing fetus.

- The list of teratogenic agents that can affect growth and development is vast and their pathological consequences can have varying degrees of severity. Moore and Persaud (2003a) gave a detailed account of these and a useful timeline of the most critical and sensitive periods of development.

- The effect of drug exposure on the developing fetus depends on several factors, such as timing of exposure, dosage, concomitant maternal disease and genetic susceptibility.

- Some infections are also known to have an adverse effect on the developing fetus (see Section 1.7).

- The causes of most common anomalies in growth and development can be categorised as malformation, disruption or deformation.

  - **Malformation** is a morphological defect that results from an intrinsically abnormal developmental process, such as a chromosomal abnormality.

  - **Disruption** occurs when there is an interference with an originally normal developmental process, as in exposure to drugs or viruses; for example, congenital amputation of an extremity or a facial cleft caused by amniotic bands (a disruption cannot be inherited).

  - **Deformation** is usually the result of mechanical forces that affect the form, shape or position of a body part, such as equinovarus foot (Moore and Persaud 2003b).

ESSENTIALS OF MIDWIFERY CARE Many factors can affect the growth and development of the fetus and it is important that the midwife is aware of this when assessing risk and planning care.

- Women with pre-existing medical conditions that require medication need urgent referral to obstetric and specialist members of the multidisciplinary team. Ideally, these women should seek pre-conceptual care as some medications are known teratogens.

- It is essential that clinicians use correct terminology when referring to fetal growth. Small for gestational age and fetal growth restriction are not the same:

  - Fetuses with a weight <10th percentile are not necessarily growth restricted – they may be healthy but constitutionally small.

  - Weight >10th percentile does not necessarily indicate 'normal' fetal growth. The fetus may undergo a pathological decline but still remain above the 10th percentile. The term fetal growth restriction is then appropriate.

○ The introduction of individualised growth charts has, to some extent, aided clarity in terms of the progression of normal growth (Zhang *et al.* 2010).

PROFESSIONAL ACCOUNTABILITY

- Timely and appropriate referral is essential if there are any concerns regarding fetal growth and development. Accurate, contemporaneous documentation should reflect all care and referrals.
- The midwife should have a good understanding of screening and diagnostic procedures available and the different methods employed to monitor fetal health.
- Midwives are required to facilitate, respect and support maternal choice.
- The midwife should be aware of relevant legislation regarding human fertilisation and embryology.

Further Resources

Pardi, G. and Cetein, I. (2006) Human fetal growth and organ development: 50 years of discoveries. *American Journal of Obstetrics and Gynecology*, **194** (4), 1088–1099.

This interesting paper discusses developments in our knowledge of intrauterine growth and development over the past 50 years. It focuses on a 'progressive walk backwards' in terms of a deeper understanding of anatomy, function and fetal diseases.

Gestational Diabetes Mellitus

Gestational diabetes mellitus (GDM) is defined as any degree of glucose intolerance that is first diagnosed during pregnancy. Its diagnosis may represent previously undiagnosed type 1 or type 2 diabetes and may predispose women to type 2 diabetes later in life (Mielke *et al.* 2013). Diagnosis of GDM places women in a higher risk category, requiring care from a multidisciplinary team. Although NICE (2014b) antenatal care guidelines do not recommend routine testing for glycosuria, screening for gestational diabetes and assessment of risk factors are recommended.

KEY POINTS

- Maternal physiological changes to ensure fetal growth and development, the transition to extrauterine life and to meet increasing maternal demands require major changes in metabolic processes and endocrine function.

- Human placental lactogen (hPL), oestrogen and progesterone in particular influence metabolic changes by altering glucose utilisation and insulin action. These changes contribute to the diabetogenic effects of pregnancy and can predispose to GDM (Blackburn 2013).

- Pregnancy causes an increase in insulin resistance resulting in altered glucose metabolism. Women with GDM also have decreased numbers of insulin receptors and decreased binding of insulin to target cells, which result in a progressive alteration in glucose tolerance (Blackburn 2013).

- GDM commonly manifests from 20 weeks' gestation when increasing levels of placental hormones block the body's ability to use insulin effectively (Wylie and Bryce 2008; Robson and Waugh 2013).

- Glycosuria is a poor predictor of GDM and usually reflects the hyperfiltration which occurs in pregnancy (Robson and Waugh 2013).

- Diagnosis of GDM is made by an oral glucose tolerance test (a drink containing 75 g of glucose is given and blood samples are taken).

- Gestational diabetes is diagnosed if the woman has either:
  - a fasting plasma glucose level of 5.6 mmol/l or above; or
  - a 2-hour plasma glucose level of 7.8 mmol/l or above (NICE 2015b).

- Poor blood glucose control throughout pregnancy will increase the risk of fetal macrosomia, shoulder dystocia and trauma during birth for the woman and her baby; also, induction of labour and/or caesarean section, neonatal hypoglycaemia and perinatal death.

- Mielke *et al.* (2013) identified that women with GDM experience intensive monitoring during pregnancy, yet often felt that concern for their health and that of their newborn dissipated soon after giving birth.

ESSENTIALS OF MIDWIFERY CARE NICE (2015a) offers a number of recommendations for the care and support of women, including:

- Risk factors for gestational diabetes should be determined at the booking appointment. These include:
  - BMI >30 kg/m^2;
  - previous macrosomic baby weighing 4.5 kg or above;
  - previous gestational diabetes;
  - first-degree relative with diabetes;
  - family origin with a high prevalence of diabetes (South Asian, Black Caribbean and Middle Eastern).

- Women need to be fully informed of the risks associated with gestational diabetes in order to make decisions about their care.
- Offer early self-monitoring of blood glucose or a 2-hour 75 g oral glucose tolerance test (OGTT) at 16–18 weeks to test for gestational diabetes if the woman has had gestational diabetes previously, followed by OGTT at 28 weeks if the first test is normal.
- Offer an OGTT at 24–28 weeks if the woman has any other risk factors.
- Some women with GDM will respond well to lifestyle changes; for example, a low glycaemic diet and exercise may help minimise the increase in insulin resistance.
- Women with a BMI >27 kg/m^2 should be encouraged and supported to lose weight.
- Oral hypoglycaemic agents or insulin therapy may be needed if diet and exercise do not control and maintain blood glucose targets over a period of 1–2 weeks.
- Extra monitoring and care may be needed during pregnancy (and labour). If an ultrasound scan shows incipient fetal macrosomia, then hypoglycaemic therapy should be considered for women with gestational diabetes.
- All women will need referral to the multidisciplinary team, including a dietician and specialist midwife/nurse, who will advise the woman regarding self-monitoring of blood glucose and individualise targets for blood glucose and regimes/doses of hypoglycaemic therapy.
- The midwife plays a key role within the multidisciplinary team to ensure that information regarding the normal aspects of a pregnancy is not lost within a medical model of care (Abayomi *et al.* 2013).
- Ensure that the woman has contact details should she become unwell or have concerns about fetal movements.
- Psychological support and advice should be offered and any reassurance should be realistic.

PROFESSIONAL ACCOUNTABILITY

- Regular communication with the woman and the multidisciplinary team is essential for effective care.
- The NMC Code (NMC 2015) requires midwives and nurses to communicate effectively and urges us to *take reasonable steps to meet people's language and communication needs*. This is particularly pertinent given that one of the risk factors is family origin and some women may not have English as their first language.
- Midwives must ensure that care is evidence based and that they are familiar with national and local guidelines.
- All care plans, including those for birth, should be made in partnership with the woman and documented in her notes.

Further Resources

NHS Choices. *Diabetes and Pregnancy*,
    http://www.nhs.uk/conditions/pregnancy-and-baby/pages/diabetes-pregnant.aspx#close.

Infections in Pregnancy

Pregnancy poses a significant immunological challenge to the mother's immune system. Although most women are not immunocompromised, suppression of cell-mediated immunity means that some infections are a cause for concern and can place the woman, fetus and neonate at increased risk (Blackburn 2013). Routine screening for some infections in pregnancy is therefore recommended by NICE (2014b) and the Department of Health (DOH 2014).

NICE (2014b) recommends routine infection screening in early pregnancy for hepatitis B virus, HIV, rubella susceptibility and syphilis. Screening for other infections such as asymptomatic bacterial vaginosis, chlamydia, cytomegalovirus, hepatitis C, group B streptococcus and toxoplasmosis is not routinely offered, mainly due to insufficient evidence to support its clinical and cost effectiveness. However, investigation of these infections can be undertaken on an individual needs basis. The acronym TORCH (Toxoplasmosis, Other, Rubella, Cytomegalovirus and Herpes) can be used to remind midwives of some of the infections that can affect the mother and fetus. The following is an overview of these and other infections that are known to have adverse effects on the fetus, mother and the neonate (see also section 4.5).

Hepatitis B Virus (HBV)

KEY POINTS
- Hepatitis B virus is highly infectious and can be found in the blood and body fluids of infected women.
- Affecting the liver, it can cause acute and chronic illness and key complications include liver cirrhosis, liver failure and hepatocellular carcinoma (Robson and Waugh 2013).
- Hepatitis B is diagnosed by a blood test that shows a positive reaction to the hepatitis B surface antigen (HBs Ag). This indicates that the disease is highly infectious and that there is a 70–90% probability of vertical transmission (UK National Screening Committee 2010).

ESSENTIALS OF MIDWIFERY CARE NICE (2013) provides comprehensive guidance for the care of those with chronic hepatitis B. The DOH (2011) recommends hepatitis B antenatal screening and a newborn immunisation programme in their best practice guidance. A summary drawn from both is offered below to aid revision:

- Pregnant women should be offered screening so that interventions that decrease the risk of vertical transmission from mother to fetus can be offered where infection is present.
- If hepatitis B is identified, referral to an obstetrician and specialist physician, for example a hepatologist, gastroenterologist or infectious disease specialist, is required within 6 weeks of the screening test results.
- Women who book for antenatal care beyond 24 weeks' gestation should be referred immediately for clinical evaluation.
- Women should be counselled about the risks to partners and other family members.
- Women should be aware of the importance of vaccination for the baby and that a four-dose regime is required: the first dose within 24 hours of birth, then one at 1 month, at 2 months and at 1 year.
- Woman should be given advice regarding breastfeeding, including abstinence of breastfeeding if nipples are cracked or bleeding (Robson and Waugh 2013).

Syphilis

KEY POINTS
- Syphilis is caused by *Treponema pallidum*, a spirochaete bacterium that enters the body through a break in the skin and is acquired by direct sexual contact.
- The progress of the infection is described in stages. The primary stage can be overlooked as chancres[3] are painless and often difficult to see (Gould and Brooker 2008).
- *Treponema pallidum* readily crosses the placental membranes early in pregnancy and therefore infection is transmitted to the fetus.
- The fetus can become infected at any stage of the disease or at any stage of pregnancy.
- Infection can cause spontaneous miscarriage, stillbirth and congenital syphilis.
- Primary maternal infection (acquired during pregnancy) almost always causes serious fetal infection. Congenital syphilis anomalies include hydrocephalis, congenital deafness, intellectual disability and abnormal teeth and bones.
- Secondary maternal infection (acquired before pregnancy) rarely results in fetal disease or anomalies.
- Appropriate treatment of the mother kills the organism and prevents transmission across the placenta.
- Early detection through screening permits prompt treatment that prevents vertical transmission.

ESSENTIALS OF MIDWIFERY CARE NICE (2014b) provides recommendations for practice that include the following:
- Screening for syphilis should be offered to all pregnant women early in pregnancy.
- A positive result does not always mean that the woman has syphilis and repeat testing may be required.
- Women who screen positive should be referred for assessment and treatment by a genitourinary specialist within the multidisciplinary team.
- Women booking late who screen positive should be referred immediately for clinical evaluation and treatment.
- Midwives and women need to be aware that the earlier the maternal infection occurs, the greater is the effect on the fetus.

HIV

KEY POINTS
- Human immunodeficiency viruses (HIV-1 and HIV-2) are ribonucleic acid (RNA) retroviruses that multiply aggressively.
- Infection of the CD4T lymphocytes (essential components of the immune system) occurs, which progressively destroys the immune system (Gould and Brooker 2008).
- This gradual deterioration in immune function leaves the body susceptible to any form of infection (Robson and Waugh 2013).
- The virus is transferred by infected blood and body fluids from one person to another and through vertical transmission from infected mothers to infants.

---

[3] Common name given to the painless ulcer that presents in stage 1 of the infection.

- Antibodies appear about 3 months after exposure and HIV infection usually progresses in four stages, the full manifestation of the disease being acquired immune deficiency syndrome (AIDS).
- HIV crosses the placenta, a significant route for transmission, as are mode of delivery and breastfeeding.
- Prompt HAART (highly active antiretroviral therapy) is available to prevent vertical transmission. Without treatment, there is a one in four chance the baby will become infected with HIV.
- Women who are HIV positive have a small increased risk of miscarriage, stillbirth, fetal abnormality, IUGR, low birth weight and premature delivery (Robson and Waugh 2013).

ESSENTIALS OF MIDWIFERY CARE NICE (2014b) offers some basic guidance but the need for sensitive care from a midwife that addresses all the woman's needs is essential:

- Women should be offered screening for HIV early in pregnancy because appropriate intervention can reduce mother-to-child transmission of HIV infection.
- Those women who know they are HIV positive or screen HIV positive require referral for consultant care and care from appropriate members of the multidisciplinary team.
- Women should be well informed of delivery options and be actively involved in a plan of care for delivery. Vaginal birth may be an option for women with a low viral load.
- The midwife should provide sensitive advice regarding infant feeding. Breastfeeding is not advised because of the risk of vertical transmission.

Rubella

KEY POINTS
- Rubella is caused by a togavirus and is spread by droplet infection.
- Infection is transmitted from 1 week before the symptoms develop and for up to 4 days after the rash first appears.
- The rubella virus crosses the placenta hence infection is significant in pregnancy as the virus disrupts fetal development (see Section 1.5). The risk of congenital rubella defect is high during the first 20 weeks of pregnancy particularly if contracted during the first 12 weeks of pregnancy.
- Features of congenital rubella syndrome include cataracts, cardiac defects and deafness.
- The risk of anomalies when infection occurs during the second and third trimesters is lower, although functional defects to the central nervous system and internal ear and eye may occur (Moore and Persaud 2003a).
- Babies born with congenital rubella are highly infectious and may excrete rubella virus in the urine for up to 12 months. Babies require follow-up observation as neurological disorders may not be immediately obvious (Bates 2011).

ESSENTIALS OF MIDWIFERY CARE NICE (2014b) offers some guidance but an understanding of immunological responses is useful when interpreting screening results:

- Rubella susceptibility screening should be offered to all women early in pregnancy.
- If rubella infection is suspected, a blood test should be obtained. Presence of IgM antibodies indicates a new rubella infection whereas the presence of IgG antibodies indicates past infection or immunisation. If both are absent, then this indicates neither infection nor immunity from the virus (DeSantis *et al.* 2006).
- Women who are not immune should be offered vaccination in the postnatal period.

- Women should be made aware of the risks of rubella infection in pregnancy and the infectious status of babies born with congenital rubella (Public Health England 2014).

Other Infections in Pregnancy
Chicken Pox

KEY POINTS
- Varicella zoster virus is a DNA virus of the herpes family and is responsible for chickenpox.
- It is highly contagious and is transmitted by respiratory droplets and by direct contact with vesicle fluid or indirectly via fomites such as skin cells, hair, clothing and bedding.
- The incubation period is between 1 and 3 weeks and the disease is infectious 48 hours before the rash appears and continues to be infectious until the vesicles crust over.
- Following the primary infection, the virus remains dormant but can be reactivated later in life and cause shingles.
- Pregnant women with no or uncertain history of chickenpox who have been exposed to infection should be tested to determine immunity.
- If the non-immune woman has had significant exposure, then varicella zoster immunoglobulin should be given and is effective when given up to 10 days after contact (Robson and Waugh 2013).
- Varicella infection in the pregnant woman is associated with pneumonia, hepatitis and encephalitis and, rarely, may result in death.
- The effect of maternal varicella infection on the fetus is determined by gestational age at the time of infection.
- Maternal varicella infection in the first 20 weeks of pregnancy results in congenital varicella syndrome in about 20% of neonates, causing chorioretinitis, skin lesions, skeletal abnormalities, encephalitis and neurological damage.
- Maternal infection developing within 5 days before or 2 days after delivery has serious implications because the fetus is unprotected by maternal antibodies and the viral dose is high.
- Maternal varicella pneumonia complicates 10–20% of cases of chickenpox in pregnancy (Lamont *et al.* 2011).

ESSENTIALS OF MIDWIFERY CARE The RCOG Green-top Guideline (RCOG 2015b) provides comprehensive guidance regarding care and treatment, including the following:
- Women should be asked about previous chickenpox/shingles infection at booking.
- Women who have not had chickenpox or are known to be seronegative for chickenpox should be advised to avoid contact with chickenpox or shingles during pregnancy and to inform the midwife or GP should exposure occur.
- A pregnant woman who develops chickenpox should be isolated from other pregnant women.
- Varicella vaccination is an option pre-pregnancy or postnatally for women who are found to be seronegative.
- Oral acyclovir should be prescribed for pregnant women with chickenpox if they present within 24 hours of the onset of the rash and if they are beyond 20 weeks' gestation. Before 20 weeks' gestation it should be considered with caution.
- Timing and mode of delivery must be individualised.

- Pregnant women with varicella zoster virus are at risk of pneumonia and should be hospitalised for monitoring and to initiate antiviral therapy (Lamont *et al.* 2011).
- Babies should be given varicella zoster immunoglobulin to reduce the risk of serious complications, including hepatic disorders and pneumonia.
- Acyclovir can be given to the neonate prophylactically.

Toxoplasmosis
KEY POINTS
- Toxoplasmosis is caused by the protozoan parasite *Toxoplasma gondii* and is a common parasitic infection.
- It occurs when infected meat is consumed or during contact with infected pets or livestock. Cats frequently harbour *T. gondii* (Gould and Brooker 2008) and their faeces can contaminate soil for up to 18 months (Robson and Waugh 2013).
- Infection is usually asymptomatic or may result in mild flu-like symptoms.
- The *T. gondii* organism crosses the placenta and infects the fetus, causing destructive changes in the brain and eye and other anomalies (Moore and Persaud 2003a).
- The risk of adverse outcome is highest following exposure in the first trimester of pregnancy. First and second trimester infection can cause miscarriage; third trimester infection can cause stillbirth.
- Clinical signs of neonatal toxoplasmosis include low birth weight, enlarged spleen and liver, hydrocephalus, jaundice and anaemia.
- A large percentage of congenitally infected infants will be asymptomatic at birth but many will develop complications including seizures and reduced cognitive function over time (Bates 2011).
- Diagnosis can be confirmed by history of clinical symptoms and antibody testing.

ESSENTIALS OF MIDWIFERY CARE NICE (2014b) guidelines do not recommend routine antenatal serological screening for toxoplasmosis. However, they advise that pregnant women should be informed of primary prevention measures:
- Midwives need to advise women to seek medical advice if they feel unwell as symptoms can be mistaken for other illness.
- Women should be aware that infection can also be asymptomatic.
- Midwives should inform women how the infection can be acquired and to take all reasonable precautions, such as:
  o hand washing;
  o thoroughly washing all fruit and vegetables;
  o cooking all raw and ready prepared meals thoroughly;
  o wearing gloves and thoroughly washing hands after gardening;
  o avoiding cat faeces in cat litter or in soil.
- Referral to the multidisciplinary team for advice on treatment is required where infection is present. Spiramycin can be used to reduce the risk of transmission of the infection. Other medication is required if tests reveal fetal infection (Robson and Waugh 2013).

Listeriosis
KEY POINTS
- Listeriosis is caused by the Gram-positive bacillus *Listeria monocytogenes*.
- It is a food-borne pathogen found throughout the environment in soil and water and also on vegetation.

- Most people develop immunity through exposure to the bacteria in the environment and some are asymptomatic carriers.
- Infection occurs with consumption of contaminated food and the incubation period is 7–70 days.
- Infection in pregnancy may be asymptomatic or women may develop flu-like symptoms.
- *Listeria* crosses the placenta and can cause spontaneous miscarriage, pre-term labour, amnionitis, stillbirth or delivery of an acutely ill baby.
- Neonatal listeriosis is classified as early or late onset. In early onset the infant has a widespread rash with septicaemia, pneumonia and meningitis. With late-onset listeriosis, meningitis is the most common presentation.
- Diagnosis is made by blood, placenta or liquor cultures and it can be treated with penicillin and erythromycin (Stables 2010; Bates 2011; Robson and Waugh 2013).

ESSENTIALS OF MIDWIFERY CARE
- There is no routine screening for listeriosis in the United Kingdom.
- Women should be advised to seek medical advice if they develop any flu-like symptoms.
- Midwives need to make women aware of the causes and risks associated with listeria.
- Women should be given information about the possible sources of infection.
- Consumption of unpasteurised milk, including milk products, brie, camembert and blue vein cheese, undercooked chicken and prepared salads such as coleslaw should be avoided.
- Food hygiene and storage are essential as *Listeria* grows at temperatures as low as 2°C and multiplies in refrigerated food and at temperatures up to 40°C (Gould and Brooker 2008).
- If maternal listeriosis is suspected or diagnosed, then referral for treatment together with regular monitoring of maternal and fetal well-being is required.

Cytomegalovirus
KEY POINTS
- Cytomegalovirus (CMV) belongs to the double-stranded DNA herpes family of viruses.
- It is transmitted by contact with infected blood, saliva or urine or by sexual contact (Stables 2010).
- After primary infection it remains latent but may become active if immunity is compromised.
- Infection in pregnancy crosses the placenta.
- If primary infection occurs in pregnancy it may cause abortion, pre-term labour, intrauterine growth restriction or fetal death.
- The greatest risk to the fetus is within the first 20 weeks of pregnancy. The virus may damage the fetal liver and nervous system.
- Clinical signs and symptoms associated with congenital CMV include microcephaly, cerebral palsy, pneumonitis, jaundice, thrombocytopenia and viral shedding.
- A small proportion of infants with congenital CMV will develop one or more physical or mental problems later in life, including hearing loss, visual impairment and learning difficulties.
- Neonatal infection occurs in two thirds of infants born by vaginal delivery.
- CMV can pass via breast milk; however, the benefits of breastfeeding outweigh the risk. One exceptional circumstance is prematurity (Bates 2011).

ESSENTIALS OF MIDWIFERY CARE

- Women should be advised to seek medical advice if they develop any flu-like symptoms.
- Midwives need to make women aware of the causes and risks associated with CMV.
- Midwives can endorse good levels of hygiene such as hand washing before preparing and eating food, before and after going to the toilet and after changing a baby's nappy.

Herpes Simplex Virus

KEY POINTS

- Herpes simplex virus (HSV) is a DNA virus responsible for cold sores and genital ulceration. HSV-1 is primarily isolated from oral lesions and HSV-2 is primarily isolated from genital lesions (Gould and Brooker 2008).
- Following primary infection the virus remains dormant. Reactivation can be provoked by stress and viral infections.
- The virus is spread by close personal contact, kissing or sexual contact.
- Some women show no clinical signs of infection, with diagnosis made following the appearance of neonatal infection acquired during birth.
- Intrauterine infection during the first 20 weeks of pregnancy can lead to miscarriage, stillbirth and congenital anomalies characterised by skin vesicles or scarring, eye lesions, neurological damage, growth restriction and impaired psychomotor development.
- Genital infection may lead to serious neonatal infection. An infected baby may develop localised lesions, encephalitis or generalised herpes infection, including viraemia, liver dysfunction and coagulopathy.
- Treatment should commence as soon as diagnosis is made by culture of the virus from affected skin and blood testing for specific antibodies.
- The infected neonate requires treatment with systemic acyclovir.

   (Straface et al. 2012; Robson and Waugh 2013).

ESSENTIALS OF MIDWIFERY CARE Robson and Waugh (2013) suggest that:

- A history of HSV infection should be obtained at booking and the woman should be advised to report any symptoms of genital herpes.
- Swabs should be obtained to confirm diagnosis and genitourinary referral should be part of care.
- If lesions are present within 6 weeks of delivery, blood tests should be taken to compare the presence of antibodies. If they are of the same type as isolated from the genital swab, this could confirm an episode of primary infection or recurrent origin.
- General hygiene advice and advice regarding pain relief should be given.
- Mode of delivery should be discussed.
- Counselling and support should be offered.

Erythrovirus (Parvovirus) B19

KEY POINTS

- This is also known as slapped cheek syndrome and fifth disease.
- Human parvovirus B19 is a small, single-stranded, non-enveloped DNA virus and a member of the Parvoviridae family.
- It is responsible for erythema infectiosum (fifth disease), the erythrovirus being a potent inhibitor of erythropoiesis.

- Infection usually occurs through respiratory droplets and hand-to-mouth contact but can also be transmitted by blood, blood-derived products and the placenta.
- Viraemia occurs 4–14 days after exposure and may last for up to 20 days.
- A rash may begin around day 15 by which time the person is usually no longer infectious. Many remain asymptomatic.
- Infection with parvovirus B19 during pregnancy can cause miscarriage and serious fetal complications.
- Parvovirus B19 has been associated with intrauterine death, non-immune hydrops fetalis, thrombocytopenia, myocarditis and neurological manifestations. However, there are few reports of congenital anomalies.
- The interval between maternal infection/viraemia and the occurrence of fetal hydrops is often 4–5 weeks.
- Timely intrauterine fetal transfusions may improve fetal outcomes (de Jong *et al.* 2011).

ESSENTIALS OF MIDWIFERY CARE

- Women should be made aware that parvovirus B19 can be problematic and to seek medical advice. Early referral for diagnosis, monitoring and treatment is essential in the management of complications.
- Some reassurance can be given as 50% of children over 15 years of age have detectable B19 IgG, and many women will therefore be immune.
- Midwives need to be aware that parvovirus B19-specific antibodies become detectable within 7–10 days after infection and therefore before signs are apparent (de Jong *et al.* 2011).

Streptococcal Infection

Streptococci are Gram-positive, chain-forming cocci classified by Rebecca Lancefield in 1933 into sub-groups A–S. Lancefield groups A and B are of most significance in childbearing (Gould and Brooker 2008; Robson and Waugh 2013).

Group B streptococcus (GBS)

KEY POINTS

- Group B streptococcus (GBS) or *Streptococcus agalactiae* is a commensal found in the gastrointestinal tract and vagina in 15–30% of woman in the United Kingdom (Feldman 2001).
- GBS is a common cause of meningitis, septicaemia and pneumonia in the newborn infant. Early-onset infection is defined as infection at less than 7 days of age and late-onset infection occurs between 7 and 90 days.
- Infection can occur *in utero* when the organism's enzymes make microscopic holes in the amniotic sac, allowing passage to the amniotic fluid or at delivery.
- Many women are asymptomatic carriers although it may cause urinary tract infection (Gould and Brooker 2008). Therefore, GBS is often identified through opportunistic analysis of a midstream specimen of urine and can be treated.
- Antenatal prophylaxis with oral benzylpenicillin for vaginal/rectal colonisation does not reduce the likelihood of GBS colonisation at the time of delivery.
- GBS bacteriuria is associated with a higher risk of chorioamnionitis and therefore serious maternal and neonatal morbidity.
- Intrapartum antibiotic prophylaxis (IAP) is offered to women with recognised risk factors for early-onset GBS, which include known carrier status, previous infant affected with

GBS, prematurity, prolonged rupture of membranes (>18 hours) and maternal fever during labour (>36 °C) (RCOG 2012).

ESSENTIALS OF MIDWIFERY CARE Whereas NICE (2014b) does not recommend routine antenatal screening for group B streptococcus in the United Kingdom, the RCOG (2012) offers guidelines for the prevention of early-onset neonatal group B streptococcal disease which include:

- Midwives need to be aware of the risks to the neonate and therefore timely referral is essential.
- Women presenting with GBS bacteriuria should be treated; GBS identified on a vaginal/rectal swab should not.
- If chorioamnionitis is suspected, a broad-spectrum antibiotic including an agent active against GBS should replace GBS-specific treatment and induction of labour should be considered.
- Antibiotic prophylaxis specific for GBS is not required for women undergoing planned caesarean section in the absence of labour and with intact membranes.
- Women need to be advised to contact the labour ward if they suspect pre-term labour or premature rupture of membranes.
- Immediate induction of labour is indicated for women known to be colonised who present at term with pre-labour rupture of membrane.
- Ideally intravenous antibiotics should be given for at least 4 hours prior to delivery.

ADDITIONAL EVIDENCE POINTS
- Evidence suggests that most hepatitis B immunisation programmes fail to provide full protection for all babies at risk, partly due to the organisation of services. However, it is the uptake of immunisation doses two and four that poses most concern (UK National Screening Committee 2010).
- The British HIV Association offers extensive guidelines for the management of HIV infection in pregnant women and provides guidance on best clinical practice, including the use of antiviral therapy both to prevent mother-to-child HIV transmission and for the welfare of the mother.
- Since the introduction of the MMR vaccine in the 1980s, controversies surrounding its administration to infants may have compromised the percentage of women immune to the rubella virus (Boyle 2011). This is an important consideration as the age group that it affected are now of childbearing age.
- Rubella was the first virus demonstrated to be a teratogen (De Santis *et al.* 2006).
- Lamont *et al.* (2011) outlined the serious nature of varicella zoster virus infection in pregnancy and discussed the role of maternal varicella zoster immunoglobulin administration.
- Elbaz *et al.* (2007) assessed the awareness of both front and second-line staff of parvovirus B19 as a potential and treatable cause of hydrops fetalis. They found that there was a need for education updates on the effect of parvovirus B19 infection during pregnancy.

PROFESSIONAL ACCOUNTABILITY
- Midwives should be aware of local protocols to ensure multidisciplinary links and timely referral.
- The acceptance or declining of all screening and/or treatment should be documented.

- A contemporaneous record of the date and time of any blood samples and swabs taken should be kept. All results and subsequent care plan should be discussed and documented.
- Results should be conveyed to the woman in a sensitive and timely manner.
- The woman's infection status should be appropriately documented in her central hospital record in order to maintain confidentiality.
- Informed consent should be obtained for all aspects of care and this should be documented.
- Some infections in pregnancy can be of a sensitive nature and women need to be treated in a non-judgemental manner. The NMC Code (NMC 2015) urges midwives to treat people with dignity and this translates to empathy, compassion and intelligent kindness.

Further Resources

Health Protection Agency (2004) *"Good Practice" Recommendations for the Prevention of Early Onset Neonatal Group B Streptococcal (GBS) Infection in the UK*, http://www.blf.net/fo/uk_goodpractice_gbs.pdf.

British HIV Association. *Clinical Guidelines*, http://www.bhiva.org/guidelines.aspx.

Public Health England (2014) *Immunisation Against Infectious Disease. The Green Book*, https://www.gov.uk/government/collections/immunisation-against-infectious-disease-the-green-book.

Intrahepatic Cholestasis of Pregnancy

Intrahepatic cholestasis of pregnancy (ICP), also referred to as obstetric cholestasis (OC), is a common form of liver disease unique to pregnancy and is associated with significant perinatal mortality and maternal morbidity. It is characterised by otherwise unexplained pruritus, elevated transaminases and bile acids in the late second half and third trimester of pregnancy, although it has been reported as early as 6–10 weeks' gestation in multiple pregnancies. The exact pathophysiology of ICP is unknown but genetic, endocrine and environmental factors are implicated (Wickström Shemer et al. 2013).

KEY POINTS

- ICP is defined as an impairment or cessation of bile flow. Bile acids are a major constituent of bile, hence any degree of suppression leads to a reduction in clearance of bile acids.

- Accumulation of bile acids within the liver increases bile acid levels which may cause widespread pruritus. When the itching involves the palms of the hands and soles of the feet and is typically worse at night, this is particularly suggestive of obstetric cholestasis.

- Differential diagnosis is determined by exclusion of other causes of pruritus and abnormal LFTs, for example, hepatitis A, B and C, biliary cirrhosis, gallbladder disease, duct dilatation and other liver pathology.

- The causal role of oestrogens is unclear; however, the manifestation of IPC in the third trimester when oestrogen levels are high and in multiple pregnancies when oestrogen concentrations are elevated imply a cholestatic response to high levels of oestrogens. Progesterone metabolites have also been implicated in the aetiopathogenesis of ICP (Vallejo et al. 2006).

- Women with IPC may experience insomnia, fatigue, depression, upper right quadrant discomfort, nausea, vomiting, weight loss and jaundice. Malabsorption of fat-soluble vitamin K can predispose to postpartum haemorrhage.

- Fetal compromise is caused by an increase in the flow of bile from the mother to the fetus together with a reduced ability of the fetus to eliminate toxic bile acids synthesised by its own liver (bile acids are synthesised by the fetal liver from around 12 weeks).

- Bile acid levels above 40 μmol/l are associated with an increased incidence of meconium-stained liquor. Geenes et al. (2013) identified a significant correlation between maternal serum bile acid levels and adverse fetal outcomes.

- Bile acids have a dose-related effect on myometrial contractility which may explain the increased incidence of spontaneous pre-term labour.

- Ursodeoxycholic acid (UDCA) improves pruritus and liver function in women with IPC.

ESSENTIALS OF MIDWIFERY CARE The RCOG Green-top Guideline (RCOG 2011b) offers evidence-based recommendations for care, a summary of which is offered below to aid revision:

- Intrahepatic cholestasis of pregnancy requires referral to obstetric lead care although midwifery care and reassurance are essential.

- A thorough history of current and previous pregnancies should be obtained. Other indicators of IPC include pale stool, dark urine and jaundice.

- Midwives should have a high index of suspicion when women present with pruritus.

- Pruritus may occur for days or weeks before the development of abnormal liver function. Persistent, unexplained pruritus and normal biochemistry (LFTs) should be measured every 1–2 weeks.

- Some temporary relief from pruritus may be gained from topical emollients.

- Psychological support and advice regarding the relief of pruritus should be given.

- Discussion should take place with the woman regarding the use of vitamin K, ursodeoxy-cholic acid, elective early delivery and the increased risk of caesarean section (Gurung *et al.* 2013).
- Ultrasound and cardiotocography are not reliable methods for preventing fetal death in ICP (RCOG 2011b). Increased maternal vigilance of fetal movement patterns should be encouraged (Robson and Waugh 2013).

ADDITIONAL EVIDENCE POINTS

- Geenes *et al.* (2013) identified a significant relationship between maternal serum bile acid levels and pre-term delivery, spontaneous pre-term birth, stillbirth and meconium-stained liquor.
- Chappell *et al.* (2012) suggested that a large-scale trial is needed to test whether ursodeoxycholic acid reduces adverse perinatal outcomes.

PROFESSIONAL ACCOUNTABILITY

- Midwives should be aware of current best evidence and their local trust guidelines.
- Midwives need to be competent in their clinical and technical knowledge base in order to deliver effective care.
- A plan of care for pregnancy and birth should be made in partnership with the woman.
- All care and plans of care should be accurately documented in the notes.
- Psychological support and advice regarding the condition should be given and any reassurance should be realistic.

Minor Disorders of Pregnancy

Minor disorders of pregnancy are rarely life threatening but can be the cause of discomfort and distress for many women. Causes fall into four main categories and are in response to the growing fetus: hormonal changes, accommodation changes, metabolic changes and postural changes (Blackburn 2013). Some minor disorders are more troublesome in the early weeks of pregnancy and may disappear as pregnancy progresses. Others can be problematic for the woman throughout pregnancy. Most body systems are affected by the demands of the growing fetus; however, many common disorders are linked to pregnancy adaptations to the digestive system and these are the primary focus below.

KEY POINTS

- **Nausea and vomiting** (N and V) affect 50–80% of pregnant women and are usually a self-limiting disorder caused by rising levels of human chorionic gonadotrophin, oestrogens and possibly thyroxine. N and V can begin as early as 2–3 weeks and usually resolve by 10–12 weeks. A few women will develop severe vomiting (hyperemesis gravidarum), which causes dehydration, electrolyte imbalance and significant weight loss (Blackburn 2013).

- **Heartburn** affects up to 80% of pregnant women and is caused by reflux of gastric acid into the lower oesophagus. Increasing levels of progesterone relax the lower oesophageal sphincter and pressure from the growing uterus increases intragastric pressure. It usually begins in the second trimester, intensifying as pregnancy progresses, and is exacerbated by multiple pregnancy, hydramnios, obesity and bending over (Blackburn 2013).

- **Constipation** affects many pregnant women and has a tendency to be worse in the first and third trimesters. Increased levels of progesterone cause relaxation of smooth muscle and reduced peristalsis. This decrease of motility and therefore a prolonged transit time increase electrolyte and water absorption in the large intestine, resulting in a dryer, bulkier stool (Yerby 2010b).

- **Haemorrhoids** in pregnancy are caused by the relaxing effect of progesterone on the veins of the anus and a reduction in venous return due to pressure from the growing uterus. This results in stasis of blood flow, venous congestion and engorgement of the haemorrhoidal veins. Haemorrhoids are usually mild but can cause pain and intermittent bleeding from the anus (Yerby 2010b).

- **Varicose veins** may occur in the legs and vulva and are a consequence of the effect of progesterone on the smooth muscle of blood vessels walls. Pressure from the gravid uterus also causes pelvic congestion and poor venous return, resulting in vulval varicosities (Bharj and Henshaw 2011).

- **Vaginal discharge** in pregnancy is common and may contribute to the inhibition of pathogenic colonisation of the vagina. However, other vaginal discharge may be the result of infection, including:
  - *bacterial vaginosis*, which is a white–grey, fishy smelling discharge, caused by an overgrowth of bacteria;
  - *trichomoniasis*, which is a common sexually transmitted infection that manifests as a green–yellow, frothy discharge with an unpleasant smell and is associated with dysuria;
  - *Candida albicans*, which is a fungus that can cause a thick or watery discharge that may smell of yeast (Bharj and Henshaw 2011).

- **Back and pelvic** pain affects up to 70% of women. The cause is usually attributed to the effect of relaxin and progesterone on the symphysis pubis ligaments and lumbosacral joints. As pregnancy progresses, postural changes occur to counterbalance the exaggerated curvature of the lower spine caused by the increasing weight of the gravid uterus (Bharj and Henshaw, 2011).

- Other physiological changes within the body systems predispose to a range of minor disorders, including gingivitis, pica, ptyalism, leg cramps, carpel tunnel syndrome, pelvic girdle pain, fatigue, fainting and frequency of micturition (Yerby 2010b; Bharj and Henshaw 2011).

ESSENTIALS OF MIDWIFERY CARE NICE (2014b) offers a number of recommendations for the management of common symptoms of pregnancy that include the following advice and guidance for midwives and other healthcare professionals:

- **Nausea and vomiting**: The midwife can give some reassurance that N and V are not usually associated with poor pregnancy outcomes. It is possible that some degree of food aversion occurs naturally to minimise fetal exposure to toxins. Effective interventions include ginger, P6 (wrist) acupressure and/or antihistamines. A history of persistent vomiting, feeling unwell and ketonuria is indicative of hyperemesis gravidarum. Hospital admission is required for intravenous fluid therapy to correct fluid and electrolyte imbalance.

- **Heartburn**: Advice regarding lifestyle and diet modifications can be given by the midwife. This includes sleeping propped up and assuming an upright position after meals, reducing food with a high fat content and avoiding other gastric irritant foods. When lifestyle and diet modifications fail to relieve symptoms, antacids may be considered.

- **Constipation**: Lifestyle and diet modifications form the greater part of midwifery advice. Adequate intake of fluids, inclusion of bran or wheat fibre supplementation and a diet rich in fruits and vegetables together with regular exercise may preclude the need for aperients.

- **Haemorrhoids:** These occur frequently in pregnancy and can be aggravated by constipation. Measures taken for the avoidance of constipation apply to those women with haemorrhoids. Standard haemorrhoid creams can be advised but corrective treatment is usually deferred until after the birth of the baby.

- **Varicose veins**: Women are advised to avoid standing for long periods, to exercise leg muscles, to elevate the legs and to wear compression stockings to improve symptoms. Vulval varicosities are rare but very painful. Women may gain some relief from the counter pressure of a substantial sanitary pad. Care must be taken during the birth as the distended veins can haemorrhage or be cut during episiotomy.

- **Vaginal discharge**: An increase in vaginal discharge is common, so it is essential to determine the cause by taking vaginal or cervical swabs and refer to genito-urinary medicine clinics where indicated. If vaginal candidiasis is identified, topical treatment with imidazole can be effective; however, oral treatment for vaginal candidiasis is not recommended.

- **Backache:** Women should be advised to stand tall, with their weight evenly distributed on both legs. Lifting should be kept to a minimum and when lying down a lateral position is recommended. Exercise in water and massage are also recommended.

PROFESSIONAL ACCOUNTABILITY
- When women present with seemingly minor disorders of pregnancy it is essential that the midwife makes a differential diagnosis to exclude pathology.

- If pathology is suspected, then prompt referral to an appropriate member of the multidisciplinary team should be made and clearly documented.

- Midwives need to have an empathetic approach to care and when women choose not to make lifestyle changes, the midwife is still required to treat them with respect, dignity and compassion.

Pre-conceptual Health

Pre-conceptual care involves the provision of advice and support for women and their partners about the health strategies that maximise the likelihood of experiencing a healthy pregnancy and giving birth to a healthy baby. Of course, many women do not plan their pregnancies and therefore do not access formalised pre-conceptual services, or such services may not exist. Opportunistic health promotion that sits broadly within the *Making Every Contact Count* framework (MECC 2012) should therefore be utilised wherever possible by healthcare professionals who have regular contact with women of childbearing age, for example, in contraception and sexual health services.

KEY POINTS NICE (2012) suggests that effective pre-conception care can have a significant impact on subsequent pregnancy and birth by:

- Early recognition and prompt management of pre or coexisting maternal health problems that are associated with increased risk, for example, mental health problems, hypertension, epilepsy or sickle cell disease.
- Identifying women at increased risk. The NHS Quality Outcome Framework has previously specified that women of childbearing age should receive annual, disease-specific advice relevant to childbearing. In the 2014 MBRRACE report, Knight *et al*. (2014) recommend that women with pre-existing medical conditions should have pre-pregnancy counselling by healthcare professionals with experience of managing their disorder in pregnancy.
- Offering lifestyle advice to reduce or avoid hazardous behaviours, such as smoking, drinking excessive alcohol or substance use.
- Identifying couples who are at increased risk of having a baby with a genetic condition or chromosomal abnormality and providing them with sufficient knowledge to make informed decisions.

ESSENTIALS OF MIDWIFERY CARE NICE (2012) suggests that healthcare professionals, including midwives, offer pre-conception advice based on the following:

- The time it may take to become pregnant. If 100 couples have regular (every 2–3 days), unprotected sexual intercourse:
  - 84 will conceive within 1 year.
  - 92 will conceive within 2 years (HFEA 2010).
- Folic acid.
- **Smoking:**
  - In the 2014 MBRRACE report (Knight *et al*. 2014), almost one-quarter of the women who died had smoked during pregnancy.
  - The impact of smoke-free legislation in England is associated with a significant reduction in perinatal and infant mortality (Been *et al*. 2015).
- Illicit drug use.
- Hazardous substances or radiation.
- Vitamin A and over-the-counter medicines.
- Cervical screening.
- Immunisations.
- Previous miscarriage(s).
- Chromosome abnormalities.

- **Being overweight or obese:**
  - ○ Midwives and other health professionals should utilise any appropriate opportunity to provide women with a BMI of 30 or more with information about the health benefits of losing weight before conceiving. This should include information on the increased health risks of obesity to themselves and their unborn child.
  - ○ Midwives should share this information with tact and sensitivity – obesity is often stigmatised within Western society.
  - ○ Women with a BMI of 30 or more should be encouraged and receive committed support to reduce weight before becoming pregnant. A weight loss of 5–10% would have significant health benefits and may increase the likelihood of conceiving.
  - ○ Women should be offered specific dietary advice in preparation for pregnancy, including the need to take daily folic acid supplements (NICE 2010).

- **Alcohol consumption:**
  - ○ When planning a pregnancy, women should be advised that it is probably the safest choice not to drink alcohol at all. Either partner consuming over six units per day reduces the chance of conception.
  - ○ There is currently a lack of robust evidence around what constitutes a 'safe' amount of alcohol to consume during pregnancy, making it difficult for midwives to advise women accordingly.
  - ○ Drinking alcohol during the first trimester is not advisable because of the risk of miscarriage (RCOG 2015a).

Further Resources

Family Planning Association leaflet *Planning a Pregnancy*,
     http://www.fpa.org.uk/help-and-advice/planning-pregnancy.

An Implementation Guide and Toolkit for Making Every Contact Count,
     https://www.england.nhs.uk/wp-content/uploads/2014/06/mecc-guid-booklet.pdf.

Pre-eclampsia

Pre-eclampsia is a pregnancy-specific condition defined as new hypertension presenting after 20 weeks' gestation with significant proteinuria (NICE 2011). Although Knight *et al.* (2014) reported a significant decrease in the number of deaths from pre-eclampsia and eclampsia, the condition remains a major cause of maternal and fetal mortality and morbidity (Robson and Waugh 2013).

Many of the improvements in maternal and neonatal outcomes are due to differential diagnosis of pre-eclampsia from other hypertensive disorders and therefore appropriate management and care:

- Pre-eclampsia may be superimposed on chronic hypertension. Chronic hypertension is present at booking or before 20 weeks, for which women may already be taking antihypertensive medication.

- Pregnancy-induced/gestational hypertension is new hypertension occurring in the second half of pregnancy but without significant proteinuria.

KEY POINTS

- Pre-eclampsia is a multisystem disorder characterised by hypertension and proteinuria. It can progress to severe pre-eclampsia and eclampsia (see Section 2.7) or a variant known as HELLP[4] syndrome, which involves abnormal liver function and thrombocytopenia (RCOG 2010; Blackburn 2013).

- The exact aetiology is complex, although altered physiology explains the pathophysiology and many causative theories. These include:
  - abnormal implantation;
  - ischaemia;
  - endothelial cell damage;
  - platelet, immunological and genetic theories.

- Placental and maternal factors interact in the development of pre-eclampsia. The underlying mechanism for the development of pre-eclampsia is thought to be impaired trophoblastic invasion and adaptation of spiral arteries, resulting in a limited supply of blood to the placenta (Blackburn 2013).

- Conditions where oxygen demand is increased (e.g. multiple pregnancy) or when oxygen transfer is decreased (e.g. diabetes) predispose to pre-eclampsia.

- As demand increases during fetal growth, blood supply is insufficient. The placenta becomes ischaemic, releasing more substances that are toxic to the maternal body, in particular the circulatory system (Blackburn 2013).

- Impaired placental perfusion is also thought to result in the ischaemic placenta releasing inflammatory factors that cause platelet activation and endothelial dysfunction (Poon *et al.* 2010). Endothelial cell injury is a common feature of pre-eclampsia.

- Increased systemic vascular resistance occurs, which causes an increase in blood pressure, resulting in decreased perfusion of most organs.

- These characteristics can culminate in maternal renal and liver failure, liver rupture, intracerebral bleeds, disseminated intravascular coagulation (DIC) and death.

- An immunological basis for pre-eclampsia is supported by the increased frequency of pre-eclampsia in first pregnancies where the mother's system responds to paternal antigens expressed on fetal tissues. This can also occur in the multigravida woman who has a new partner (Williams and Broughton Pipkin 2011; Blackburn 2013).

---

[4] Haemolysis (H), elevated liver enzymes (EL) and low platelet count (LP).

- Fetal complications include growth restriction, prematurity, placental abruption, hypoxia and intrauterine death (Blackburn 2013; Robson and Waugh, 2013).

ESSENTIALS OF MIDWIFERY CARE NICE (2011, 2014b) makes the following recommendations for the care and support of women:

- At booking, the following risk factors for pre-eclampsia should be determined:
  - age 40 years or older;
  - nulliparity;
  - pregnancy interval of more than 10 years;
  - family history of pre-eclampsia (including paternal family history);
  - previous history of pre-eclampsia;
  - body mass index 30 kg/m^2 or more;
  - pre-existing vascular disease such as hypertension;
  - pre-existing renal disease;
  - multiple pregnancy.
- Women who have more than one moderate risk factor for pre-eclampsia should be advised to take 75 mg of aspirin daily from 12 weeks until the birth of the baby.
- All pregnant women should be made aware of the need to seek immediate advice from a healthcare professional if they experience symptoms of pre-eclampsia. These include:
  - severe headache;
  - problems with vision, such as blurring or flashing before the eyes;
  - severe pain just below the ribs;
  - vomiting;
  - sudden swelling of the face, hands or feet.
- Midwives should ensure that the woman is aware of symptoms which need immediate clinical review.
- Blood pressure measurements and urinalysis for protein should be carried out at each antenatal visit to screen for pre-eclampsia.
- The degree of hypertension will determine care management:
  - mild hypertension = 140/90 to 149/99 mmHg;
  - moderate hypertension = 150/100 to 159/109 mmHg;
  - severe hypertension = 160/110 mmHg or higher.
- Hypertension where there is a single diastolic blood pressure of 110 mmHg or two consecutive readings of 90 mmHg at least 4 hours apart and/or significant proteinuria (1+) should prompt consultant referral and increased surveillance.
- If the systolic blood pressure is above 160 mmHg on two consecutive readings at least 4 hours apart, treatment should be considered.
- Korotkoff phase 5 is the appropriate measurement of diastolic pressure. The method used should be consistent and documented. Automated methods should be used with caution.
- Significant proteinuria equates to more than 300 mg of protein in a 24-hour urine collection or more that 30 mg/mmol in a spot urinary protein/creatinine sample.
- Blood samples should be taken for analysis and include urea and electrolytes, LFTs, full blood count and serum creatinine. These should be measured against a reference range specific to pregnancy:

- ° urea and electrolytes and serum creatinine indicate kidney function;
- ° a full blood count indicates platelet consumption, haemolysis and haemoconcentration;
- ° liver enzymes such as transaminases and bilirubin indicate liver function.
- Women diagnosed with severe gestational hypertension or pre-eclampsia require fetal monitoring. This should include cardiotocography, ultrasound fetal growth and amniotic volume assessment and umbilical artery Doppler velocimetry.
- Assessment should be performed by a healthcare professional trained in the management of hypertensive disorders of pregnancy. Consultant care is therefore indicated as antihypertensive medication, fetal surveillance (as above), admission or early delivery may be indicated. Corticosteroids should be given if delivery is anticipated at <34 weeks' gestation.

ADDITIONAL EVIDENCE POINTS

- Although pre-eclampsia commonly manifests at around 20 weeks, there is evidence that biophysical and biochemical markers are evident at 11–13 weeks' gestation (Poon *et al.* 2010).
- Familial clustering of pre-eclampsia suggests a genetic component. Higher rates of pre-eclampsia have been noted in pregnancies fathered by men whose mothers had pre-eclampsia (Williams and Broughton Pipkin 2011).

PROFESSIONAL ACCOUNTABILITY

- Midwives need to be competent in their clinical and technical knowledge base to deliver effective care.
- Midwives must ensure that care is timely and evidence based and that they are familiar with national and local guidelines.
- A plan of care for birth should be made in partnership with the woman and accurately documented in the notes.
- Psychological support and advice regarding the condition should be given and any reassurance should be realistic.

Further Resources

Action on Pre-eclampsia (APEC). *Midwives E-Learning Presentation*,
    http://action-on-pre-eclampsia.org.uk/midwives-e-learning-presentation/.

Preparation for Parenthood

Traditionally known as 'parentcraft' classes, preparation for parenthood today usually takes the form of antenatal education sessions run by midwives or organisations such as the National Childbirth Trust (NCT). Despite a significant number of women attending antenatal classes, the evidence base about their impact in helping women and their partners prepare for childbirth and parenthood is currently weak; however, programmes may confer other benefits that require further exploration.

KEY POINTS

- Structured programmes that often reflect the information that maternity care staff wish to share, rather than seek what information women actually want, have generally replaced traditional forms of sharing childbirth knowledge.

- Classic approaches to antenatal education include Dick-Read's natural childbirth approach based on inhibiting the fear/tension/pain cycle (Dick-Read 1933) and Lamaze's psychoprophylaxis model (Lamaze 1958).

- More contemporary approaches include 'active birth' (Balaskas 1992) and hypnobirthing (Mongan 2005). All of these approaches aim to utilise a woman's natural coping mechanisms driven chiefly by the synergy of labour hormones.

- Most of the current research has focused on well-educated women who occupy the middle to upper socio-economic groups, generally viewed as 'typical' attendees (Gagnon and Sandall 2007). The impact of antenatal education on other groups may be of more interest from a public health perspective, as would the perspectives of men who report feeling excluded (Smith 1996).

- There is a lack of robust evidence that explores the value of antenatal education in building support networks for women. Nolan *et al.* (2012) suggested that they may be helpful in establishing friendships amongst women during pregnancy.

ESSENTIALS OF MIDWIFERY CARE The Department of Health, in partnership with key stakeholders, has developed the *Preparation for Birth and Beyond* resource pack to help midwives deliver contemporary and effective antenatal education. The chief aim of this initiative is to reduce inequalities by supporting disadvantaged parents to give their children an optimal start to life. Some key advice for midwives delivering antenatal education includes the following:

- Thinking about antenatal education in its broadest sense, then tailoring services for local communities based on local knowledge and expertise.

- Remembering that new parents are keen for information but need time to reflect on it and therefore do not want it delivered to them all at once.

- Tailoring sessions that offer consistent information and advice.

- Involving fathers and including information specific to their needs.

- Considering the needs of women from different groups; for example, young parents often prefer to participate in peer groups.

- Offering broad-based content that does not focus just on labour and birth.

- Recognising that midwives will be at their most effective when drawing on the knowledge, experience and expertise of parents.

ADDITIONAL EVIDENCE POINTS Schrader McMillan *et al.* (2009):

- Antenatal education has a clear role to play in the education of new parents.

- Group-based antenatal programmes that cover a broad range of topics are associated with improved maternal well-being.

- Participation in group-based sessions can support women with symptoms of anxiety and depression.

PROFESSIONAL ACCOUNTABILITY

- Under Article 42 of the EU Midwifery Directive, midwives have a responsibility in the *provision of programmes of parenthood preparation and complete preparation for childbirth including advice on hygiene and nutrition.*

- Although many midwives may perceive that they lack the skills for the delivery of effective antenatal education, they have a clear responsibility under the NMC Code (NMC 2015) both to maintain their skills and to seek opportunities to develop them further. Working in partnership with women and their families to identify learning needs can be a significant factor in this regard.

Further Resources

Department of Health. *Preparation for Birth and Beyond: a Resource Pack for Leaders of Community Groups and Activities,* https://www.gov.uk/government/uploads/system/uploads/attachment_data/file/215386/dh_134728.pdf.

References

Abayomi, J., Wood, L., Spelman, S., Morrison, G. and Purewal, T. (2013) The multidisciplinary management of type 2 and gestational diabetes in pregnancy. *British Journal of Midwifery*, **21** (4), 236–242.

Balaskas, J. (1992) *Active Birth: the New Approach to Giving Birth Naturally*, Harvard Common Press, Boston, MA.

Bates, C. (2011) Infection, in *Mayes' Midwifery*, 14th edn (eds S. Macdonald and J. Magill-Cuerden), Baillière Tindall Elsevier, Edinburgh, pp. 689–698.

Been, J., Mackay, D., Millett, C., Pell, J., van Schayck, O. and Sheikh, A. (2015) Impact of smoke-free legislation on perinatal and infant mortality: a national quasi-experimental study. *Scientific Reports*, **5**, 13020.

Bhandari, S., Raja, E., Shetty, S. and Bhattacharya, S. (2014) Maternal and perinatal consequences of antepartum haemorrhage of unknown origin. *BJOG*, **121**, 44–52.

Bharj, K. and Henshaw, A. (2011) Confirming pregnancy and care of the pregnant woman, in *Mayes' Midwifery*, 14th edn (eds S. Macdonald and J. Magill-Cuerden), Baillière Tindall Elsevier, Edinburgh, pp. 411–441.

Billington, M. and Stevenson, M. (2007) Anaesthesia and resuscitation of the critically ill woman, in *Critical Care in Childbearing for Midwives* (eds M. Billington and M. Stevenson), Blackwell, Oxford, pp. 204–223.

Blackburn, S.T. (2013) *Maternal, Fetal and Neonatal Physiology: a Clinical Perspective*, 4th edn, Elsevier Saunders, Maryland Heights, MO.

Blann, A. (2006) *Routine Blood Results Explained. A Guide for Nurses and Allied Health Professionals,* M&K Update, Keswick.

Blows, W. (2012) *The Biological Basis of Clinical Observations*, 2nd edn, Routledge, London.

Boyle, M. (2011) Antenatal investigations, in *Mayes' Midwifery*, 14th edn (eds S. Macdonald and J. Magill-Cuerden), Baillière Tindall Elsevier, Edinburgh, pp. 443–454.

Brockington, I. (1998) *Motherhood and Mental Health*, Oxford University Press, Oxford.

Chappell, L., Gurung, V., Seed, P., Chambers, J.,Williamson, C. and Thornton, J. (2012) Ursodeoxycholic acid versus placebo, and early term delivery versus expectant management, in women with intrahepatic cholestasis of pregnancy: semifactorial randomised clinical trial. *BMJ*, **344**, e3799, available at http://www.bmj.com/content/344/bmj.e3799.short (accessed 26 June 2015).

Chase, A., Sohal, M., Howard, J., McCarthy, A., Layton, D. and Oteng-Ntim, E. (2010) Pregnancy outcomes in sickle cell disease: a retrospective cohort study from two tertiary centres in the UK. *Obstetric Medicine*, **3** (3), 110–112.

Coad, J. and Dunstall, M. (2012) *Anatomy and Physiology for Midwives*, 3rd edn, Churchill Living-stone Elsevier, Edinburgh.

de Jong, E., Walther, F., Kroes, A. and Oepkes, D. (2011) Parvovirus B19 infection in pregnancy: new insight and management. *Prenatal Diagnosis*, **31** (5), 419–425.

DeSantis, M., Cavailiere, A., Straface, G. and Caruso, A. (2006) Rubella infection in pregnancy. *Reproductive Toxicology*, **21** (4), 390–398.

Dick-Read, G. (1933) *Natural Childbirth*, Heinemann, London.

DOH (2011) *Hepatitis B Antenatal Screening and Newborn Immunisation Programme: Best Practice Guidance*, Department of Health, London, https://www.gov.uk/government/publications/hepatitis-b-antenatal-screening-and-newborn-immunisation-programme-best-practice-guidance (accessed 6 August 2015).

DOH (2014) *NHS Public Health Functions Agreement 2015–16: Service Specification No. 15: NHS Infectious Diseases in Pregnancy Screening Programme*, Department of Health, London, https://www.gov.uk/government/uploads/system/uploads/attachment_data/file/386275/No15_NHS_Infectious_Diseases_in_Pregnancy_Screening.pdf (accessed 21 November 2015).

Dunkel Schetter, C. and Tanner, L. (2012) Anxiety, depression and stress in pregnancy: implications for mothers, children, research and practice. *Current Opinion in Psychiatry*, **25**, 141–148.

Elbaz, W., Coyle, P., Hunter, A. and Farrag, S. (2007) Erythrovirus B19 as a potential cause of fetal hydrops: assessing awareness. *British Journal of Midwifery*, **15** (7), 440–443.

Family Nurse Partnership (2015) http://fnp.nhs.uk/ (accessed June 2015).

Feldman, R.G. (2001) Group B streptococcus. Prevention of infection in the newborn. *Practising Midwife*, **4** (3): 16–18.

Ferns, T. (2007) Shock and the critically ill woman, in *Critical Care in Childbearing for Midwives* (eds M. Billington and M. Stevenson), Blackwell, Oxford, pp. 140–166.

Gagnon, A. and Sandall, J. (2007) Individual or group antenatal education for childbirth or parenthood or both. *Cochrane Database of Systematic Reviews*, Issue 3 (Art. No.: CD002869), doi: 10.1002/14651858.CD002869.pub2.

Geenes, V., Chappell, L., Steed, P., Steer, P., Knight, M. and Williamson, C. (2013) Association of severe intrahepatic cholestasis of pregnancy with adverse pregnancy outcomes: a prospective population-based case-control study. *Hepatology*, **59** (4), 1482–1491.

Glover, V. (2014) Maternal depression, anxiety and stress during pregnancy and child outcome; what needs to be done. *Clinical Obstetrics and Gynaecology*, **28** (1), 25–35.

Gould, D. and Brooker, C. (2008) *Infection Prevention and Control: Applied Microbiology for Healthcare*, 2nd edn, Palgrave Macmillan, Basingstoke.

Gurung, V., Stokes, M., Middleton, P., Milan, S., Hague, W. and Thornton, J. (2013) Interventions for treating cholestasis in pregnancy. *Cochrane Database of Systematic Reviews*, Issue 6 (Art. No.: CD000493), doi: 10.1002/14651858.CD000493.pub2.

HFEA (2010) *Fertility Facts and Figures 2008*, Human Fertilisation and Embryology Authority, http://www.hfea.gov.uk/docs/2010-12-08_Fertility_Facts_and_Figures_2008_Publication_PDF.PDF (accessed 21 August 2015).

Hutcherson, A. (2011) Bleeding in pregnancy, in *Mayes' Midwifery*, 14th edn (eds S. Macdonald and J. Magill-Cuerden), Baillière Tindall Elsevier, Edinburgh, pp. 753–770.

Knight, M., Nair, M., Shah, A., Noor, N. and Acosta, C. (2014) Maternal mortality and morbidity in the UK 2009–12: surveillance and epidemiology, in *Saving Lives, Improving Mothers' Care – Lessons Learned to Inform Future Maternity Care from the UK and Ireland Confidential Enquiries into Maternal Deaths and Morbidity 2009–2012* (eds M. Knight, S. Kenyon, P. Brocklehurst, N. Neilson, J. Shakespeare and J.J. Kurinczuk, on behalf of MBRRACE-UK), National Perinatal Epidemiology Unit, University of Oxford, Oxford, pp. 9–26.

Lalor, J.G., Fawole, B., Alfirevic, Z. and Devane, D. (2008) *Cochrane Database of Systematic Reviews*, Issue 1 (Art. No.: CD000038), doi: 10.1002/14651858.CD000038.pub2.

Lamaze, F. (1958) *Painless Childbirth. Psychoprophylactic Method* (transl. L.R. Celestin), Burke, London.

Lamont, R., Sobel, J., Carrington, D., Mazaki-Tovi, S., Kusanovic, J., Vaisuch, E. and Romera, R. (2011) Varicella-zoster virus (chickenpox) infection in pregnancy. *BJOG*, **118** (10), 1155–1162.

Leight, K., Fitelson E., Weston, C. and Wisner, K. (2010) Childbirth and mental disorders. *International Review of Psychiatry*, **22**, 453–471.

McCormack, R., Doherty, D., Magann, E., Hutchinson, M. and Newham, J. (2008) Antenatal bleeding of unknown origin in the second half of pregnancy and pregnancy outcomes *BJOG*, **115**, 1451–1457.

MECC (2012) *Making Every Contact Count*, NHS Yorkshire and Humber, http://www .makingeverycontactcount.co.uk/ (accessed 14 August 2015).

Mielke, R.T., Kaises, D. and Centuola, R. (2013) Interconception care for women with prior gestational diabetes mellitus. *Journal of Midwifery and Woman's Health*, **58** (3) 303–312.

Mongan, M.F. (2005) *Hypnobirthing: the Mongan Method: a Natural Approach to a Safe, Easier, More Comfortable Birthing*, 3rd edn, Health Communications, Deerfield Beach, FL.

Moore, K.L. and Persaud, T.V.N. (2003a) *Before We Are Born: Essentials of Embryology and Birth Defects*, 6th edn, Saunders, Philadelphia, PA.

Moore, K.L. and Persaud, T.V.N. (2003b) *The Developing Human: Clinically Oriented Embryology*, 7th edn, Saunders, Philadelphia, PA.

NHS (2011) *NHS Sickle Cell and Thalassaemia (SCT) Screening Programme: Standards for the Linked Antenatal and Newborn Screening Programme*, http://sct.screening.nhs.uk (accessed 13 July 2015).

NICE (2010) *Weight Management Before, During and After Pregnancy*, NICE Public Health Guidance PH27, National Institute for Health and Clinical Excellence, London.

NICE (2011) *Hypertension in Pregnancy: the Management of Hypertensive Disorders During Pregnancy*, NICE Clinical Guideline CG107, National Institute for Health and Clinical Excellence, London.

NICE (2012) *Clinical Knowledge Summaries. Pre-conception: Advice and Management*, National Institute for Health and Clinical Excellence, London.

NICE (2013) *Hepatitis B (Chronic): Diagnosis and Management of Chronic Hepatitis B in Children, Young People and Adults*, NICE Clinical Guideline CG165, National Institute for Health and Care Excellence, London.

NICE (2014a) *Antenatal and Postnatal Mental Health: Clinical Management and Service Guidance*, NICE Clinical Guideline CG192, National Institute for Health and Care Excellence, London.

NICE (2014b) *Antenatal Care*, NICE Clinical Guideline CG62, National Institute for Health and Care Excellence, London.

NICE (2014c) *NICE Pathways. Antenatal Care Overview*, http://pathways.nice.org.uk/pathways/ antenatal-care (accessed 20 July 2015).

NICE (2015a) *Diabetes in Pregnancy: Management of Diabetes and Its Complications from Preconception to the Postnatal Period*, NICE Guideline NG3, National Institute for Health and Care Excellence, London.

NICE (2015b) *NICE Pathways. Diabetes in Pregnancy Overview*, http://pathways.nice.org.uk/ pathways/diabetes-in-pregnancy (accessed 9 July 2015).

NMC (2015) *The Code: Professional Standards of Practice and Behaviour for Nurses and Midwives*, Nursing and Midwifery Council, London.

Nolan, M., Mason, V., Snow, S., Messenger, W., Catling, J. and Upton, P. (2012) Making friends at antenatal classes: a qualitative exploration of friendship across the transition to motherhood. *Journal of Perinatal Education*, **21** (3), 178–185.

O'Connor, G., Heron, J., Glover, V. and the Alspac Study Team (2002) Antenatal anxiety predicts child behavioral/emotional problems independently of postnatal depression. *Journal of the American Academy of Child and Adolescent Psychiatry*, **41** (12), 1470–1477.

Pardi, G. and Cetein, I. (2006) Human fetal growth and organ development: 50 years of discoveries. *American Journal of Obstetrics and Gynecology*, **194** (4), 1088–1099.

Paterson-Brown, S. and Bamber, J. (2014) Prevention and treatment of haemorrhage, in *Saving Lives, Improving Mothers' Care – Lessons Learned to Inform Future Maternity Care from the UK and Ireland Confidential Enquiries into Maternal Deaths and Morbidity 2009–2012* (eds M. Knight, S. Kenyon, P Brocklehurst, N. Neilson, J. Shakespeare and J.J. Kurinczuk, on behalf of MBRRACE-UK), National Perinatal Epidemiology Unit, University of Oxford, Oxford, pp. 45–56.

Pavord, S., Mayers, B., Robinson,S., Allard, S., Strong, J. and Oppenheimer, C. (2012) UK guidelines on the management of iron deficiency in pregnancy. *British Journal of Haematology*, **156**, 588–600.

Poon, L., Akolekar, R., Lachmann, R., Beta, J. and Nicolaides, K. (2010) Hypertensive disorders in pregnancy: screening by biophysical and biochemical markers at 11–13 weeks. *Ultrasound in Obstetrics and Gynecology*, **35**, 662–670.

Public Health England (2014) *Immunisation Against Infectious Disease. The Green Book*, https://www.gov.uk/government/collections/immunisation-against-infectious-disease-the-green-book (Accessed 23 August 2015).

Public Health England (2015) *Fetal Anomaly Screening: Care Pathways*, https://www.gov.uk/government/publications/fetal-anomaly-screening-care-pathways (accessed 26 June 2015).

Qureshi, H., Massey, E., Kirwan, T., Davies, S., Robson, J., White, J., Jones, J. and Allard, S. (2014) BCSH guideline for the use of anti-D immunoglobulin for the prevention of haemolytic disease of the fetus and newborn. *Transfusion Medicine*, **24** (1), 8–20.

RCOG (2010) *The Management of Severe Pre-eclampsia*, Guideline No. 10(A), Royal College of Obstetricians and Gynaecologists, London.

RCOG (2011a) *Management of Sickle Cell Disease in Pregnancy*, Green-top Guideline No. 61, Royal College of Obstetricians and Gynaecologists, London.

RCOG (2011b) *Obstetric Cholestasis*, Green-top Guideline No. 43, Royal College of Obstetricians and Gynaecologists, London.

RCOG (2011c) *Reduced Fetal Movements*, Green-top Guideline No. 55, Royal College of Obstetricians and Gynaecologists, London.

RCOG (2011d) *Antepartum Haemorrhage*, Green-top Guideline No. 63, Royal College of Obstetricians and Gynaecologists, London.

RCOG (2011e) *Placenta Praevia, Placenta Praevia Accreta and Vasa Praevia: Diagnosis and Management*, Green-top Guideline No. 27, Royal College of Obstetricians and Gynaecologists, London.

RCOG (2012) *The Prevention of Early-onset Neonatal Group B Streptococcal Disease*, Green-top Guideline No. 36, Royal College of Obstetricians and Gynaecologists, London.

RCOG (2013) *The Investigation and Management of the Small-for-Gestational-Age Fetus*, Green-top Guideline No. 31, 2nd edn, Royal College of Obstetricians and Gynaecologists, London.

RCOG (2014) *Management of Beta Thalassaemia in Pregnancy*, Green-top Guideline No. 66, Royal College of Obstetricians and Gynaecologists, London.

RCOG (2015a) *Alcohol and Pregnancy*, Royal College of Obstetricians and Gynaecologists, London.

RCOG (2015b) *Chickenpox in Pregnancy*, Green-top Guideline No. 13, Royal College of Obstetricians and Gynaecologists, London.

Robson, E. and Waugh, J. (2013) *Medical Disorders in Pregnancy: a Manual for Midwives*, 2nd edn, John Wiley & Sons, Chichester.

Schrader McMillan, A., Barlow, J. and Redshaw, M. (2009) *Birth and Beyond: a Review of the Evidence About Antenatal Education*, Department of Health, London.

Segal, Z.V., Williams, J.M.G. and Teasdale, J.D. (2012) *Mindfulness-based Cognitive Therapy for Depression*, Guilford Press, New York.

Smith, N. (1996) Antenatal classes and the transition to fatherhood: a study of some fathers' views. *MIDIRS Midwifery Digest*, **9** (3), 327–330.

Stables, D. (2010) Common fetal problems, in *Physiology in Childbearing: with Anatomy and Related Biosciences*, 3rd edn (eds D. Stables and, J. Rankin), Baillière Tindall Elsevier, Edinburgh, pp. 185–196.

Stampalija, T., Gyte, G. and Alfirevic, Z. (2010) Doppler ultrasound: when and why? *Practising Midwife*, **13** (6), 12, 14–15.

Steen, M., Robinson, M., Robertson, S. and Raine, G. (2015) Pre and post survey findings from the Mind 'Building Resilience Programme for Better Mental Health: Pregnant Women and New Mothers', *Evidence Based Midwifery*, **13** (3), 92–99.

Straface, G., Selmin, A., Zanarda, V., DeSantis, M., Ercoli, A. and Scambia, G. (2012) Herpes simplex virus infection in pregnancy, *Infectious Diseases in Obstetrics and Gynecology*, **2012**, 385697.

UK National Screening Committee (2010) *Infectious Diseases in Pregnancy Screening Programme: Programme Standards*, https://www.gov.uk/government/publications/infectious-diseases-in-pregnancy-screening-programme-standards (accessed 6 August 2015).

Vallejo, M., Briz, O., Serrano, M., Monte, M. and Marrin, J. (2006) Potential role of trans-inhibition of the bile salt export pump by progesterone metabolites in the etiopathogenesis of intrahepatic cholestasis of pregnancy. *Journal of Hepatology*, **44**, 1150–1157.

van den Bergh, B. and Marcoen, A. (2004) High antenatal maternal anxiety is related to ADHD symptoms, externalizing problems, and anxiety in 8- and 9-year-olds. *Child Development*, **75**, 1085–1097.

Waugh, A. and Grant, A. (2014) *Ross and Wilson Anatomy and Physiology in Health and Illness*, 12th edn, Churchill Livingstone Elsevier, Edinburgh.

Wickström Shemer, E., Marschall, H.U., Ludvigsson, J.F. and Stephansson, O. (2013) Intrahepatic cholestasis of pregnancy and associated adverse pregnancy and fetal outcomes: a 12-year population-based cohort study. *BJOG*, **120** (6), 717–723.

Williams, P.J. and Broughton Pipkin, F. (2011) The genetics of pre-eclampsia and other hypertensive disorders of pregnancy. *Best Practice and Research. Clinical Observations and Gynaecology*, **25** (4), 405–417.

Wylie, L. and Bryce, H. (2008) *The Midwives' Guide to Key Medical Conditions: Pregnancy and Childbirth*, Churchill Livingstone Elsevier, Edinburgh.

Yang, Q., Wen, S., Phillips, K., Oppenheimer, L., Black, D. and Walker, M. (2009) Comparison of maternal risk factors between placental abruption and placenta previa. *American Journal of Perinatology*, **26** (4), 279–286.

Yerby, M. (2010a) Anaemia and clotting disorders, in *Physiology in Childbearing: with Anatomy and Related Biosciences*, 3rd edn (eds D. Stables and, J. Rankin), Baillière Tindall Elsevier, Edinburgh, pp. 447–458.

Yerby, M. (2010b) Minor disorders of pregnancy, in *Physiology in Childbearing: with Anatomy and Related Biosciences*, 3rd edn (eds D. Stables and, J. Rankin), Baillière Tindall Elsevier, Edinburgh, pp. 417–422.

Yerby, M. (2010c) Bleeding in pregnancy, in *Physiology in Childbearing: with Anatomy and Related Biosciences*, 3rd edn (eds D. Stables and, J. Rankin), Baillière Tindall Elsevier, Edinburgh, pp. 423–436.

Zhang, J., Merialdi, M., Platt, L. and Kramer, M. (2010) Defining normal and abnormal fetal growth: promises and challenges. *American Journal of Obstetrics and Gynaecology*, **202** (6): 522–528.

PART II

Labour and Birth

Rapid Midwifery, First Edition. Sarah Snow, Kate Taylor, and Jane Carpenter.
© 2016 John Wiley & Sons, Ltd. Published 2016 by John Wiley & Sons, Ltd.

First Stage of Labour

A pregnancy is considered to be at term from 37+0 to 41+6 weeks' gestation and during this time most women labour spontaneously (NICE 2008). However, prolonged pregnancy (over 42 weeks' gestation) will occur in 5–10% of all women (NICE 2008) and some women will labour prematurely. It is not fully understood what causes the onset of labour although it is thought to be multifactorial in nature (Kamel 2010).

The first stage of labour is often defined in two phases: the latent phase of labour and established first stage. NICE (2014a) defines the latent phase of labour as a period of time, not necessarily continuous, where painful contractions occur alongside cervical effacement and dilatation up to 4 cm. Established labour is defined as regular painful contractions with progressive cervical dilatation from 4 cm up to full dilatation (NICE 2014a).

KEY POINTS

- Provision of support during labour and childbirth is recognised internationally and nationally as a core role of the midwife (RCM 2012a). Current NICE guidance (NICE 2014a) states that all women should receive one-to-one care during established labour and that women should only be left on their own for short periods or at their own request. This clearly highlights the importance of continuous high-quality midwifery care and support during labour (RCM 2012a).

- The latent phase of labour can be particularly challenging for women, especially if it is long-lasting, which can be exhausting and discouraging (RCM 2012d). Good antenatal education and early assessment advice should encourage women to remain at home during the latent phase, if they feel able. Admission to hospital during the latent phase may increase intervention rates (Bailit et al. 2005).

- Evidence has shown that women who receive continuous support in labour are more likely to have spontaneous vaginal birth and less likely to require intrapartum analgesia or to be dissatisfied with the care they received (Hodnett et al. 2011). They also have shorter labours, are less likely to require operative deliveries, are less likely to require epidural analgesia and are less likely to have a baby with a low 5-minute APGAR score (Hodnett et al. 2011).

- Giving a definitive answer to the question of how long a labour will last is difficult, due not least to inaccuracies in measuring labour length (RCM 2012c). In addition, several factors can influence the length of the first stage of labour, including, but not limited to, parity (Lawrence et al. 2013), fetal position at labour onset (Simkin 2010), presence of continuous care in labour (Hodnett et al. 2011) and use of upright birth positions (Lawrence et al. 2013).

- For some women, induction or augmentation of labour may be indicated. Various methods can be used to mimic or replicate physiological labour. However, any such intervention will be associated with risk and disrupt physiological processes, making informed choice essential.

ESSENTIAL PHYSIOLOGY

- Certain hormones, notably oestrogen and progesterone, are accepted as having an important role in maintaining uterine quiescence during pregnancy and in initiating uterine activity at labour onset (Kamel 2010).

- The roles of other hormones (such as prostaglandins) and other factors (such as inflammatory reactions) are currently poorly understood. There may be yet other factors still to be discovered.

- The hormone oxytocin causes the continuation of uterine contractions via a positive feedback loop. If this loop is broken, contractions will be disrupted (Chapman and Charles 2013).

- Oxytocin is often referred to as a 'shy hormone'. In order to promote oxytocin release, women should feel safe, secure and supported (Westbury 2015). Feelings of stress or panic cause the release of catecholamines which, in turn, inhibit oxytocin; whereas oxytocin itself encourages the release of endorphins (Westbury 2015). It is a key part of the midwife's role to enable oxytocin release by creating a sense of privacy, calm and safety.

- Uterine contractions during the first stage of labour cause effacement (thinning or shortening of the cervical length) and dilatation (opening) of the cervix; they also aid fetal descent into the pelvis:
  - In normal uterine action, contractions begin in the cornua of the uterus and spread downwards. This is known as fundal dominance.
  - The upper segment of the uterus contracts and retracts powerfully, whereas the lower segment contracts only slightly but dilates.
  - The coordination between the upper and lower uterine segments is balanced during normal labour and is known as polarity.
  - The uterus has a low resting tone between contractions, which is essential for fetal oxygenation (Walsh 2011).

- For a nulliparous woman, the cervix may not begin to dilate until it is fully (100%) effaced. For parous women, however, effacement and dilatation may occur simultaneously. Full dilatation is reached at about 10 cm.

- Women may experience a 'show' as their cervix dilates. This 'operculum' forms a mucus plug over the cervix during pregnancy. The mucoid show may contain streaks of bloody discharge; however, fresh red blood loss is not a normal part of a show.

- As the fetus descends through the cervix, it separates the small bag of membranes in front, the forewaters, from the remainder that follows behind, the hindwaters:
  - The forewaters aid effacement and early dilatation of the cervix.
  - The hindwaters help to equalize uterine pressure, thereby offering some protection for the fetus and placenta (Walsh 2011).

- At some point during labour, the membranes surrounding the amniotic fluid will rupture. Prior to this bulging, forewaters can often be felt on vaginal examination (Chapman and Charles 2013).

- Spontaneous rupture of membranes normally occurs towards the end of the first stage of labour (RCM 2015b). This can lead to stronger application of the fetal head to the cervix during contractions, intensifying the positive feedback loop and leading to transition and the second stage of labour.

- The membranes can also rupture before labour onset or during the second stage, or rarely a baby can be born within the amniotic sac.

ESSENTIALS OF MIDWIFERY CARE

- Women should be encouraged to write down their birth preferences prior to labour onset. If this has been done, these should be read and discussed with the woman and her birth partner.

- It is important to listen to and understand a woman's preferences for pain relief during labour and to support her in her choices (NICE 2014a).

- A woman's chosen birth partners have an important role to play, providing emotional support and advocacy. They should be included in discussions of birth options and be encouraged to provide practical support tasks where appropriate (RCM 2012e).

- Alongside the emotional support provided, continuous assessment of maternal and fetal well-being is another essential component of a midwife's role during established labour. NICE (2014a) summarises this as follows:
  - Ongoing consideration of a woman's desire for pain relief, including enabling her to request pain relief at any point during labour.
  - Encouragement to stay well hydrated. A light diet should be supported if the woman desires.
  - Auscultation of the fetal heart rate. For low-risk women this should be carried out for 1 minute immediately after a contraction, using either a Pinard stethoscope or Doppler ultrasound. Accelerations and decelerations should be recorded if heard.
  - Continuous electronic fetal monitoring should be used only if indicated. Telemetry can be used to enable active labour and birth.
  - Maternal observations should be recorded and documented on a partogram, including:
    - the frequency of contractions half-hourly;
    - hourly pulse;
    - 4-hourly temperature and blood pressure;
    - frequency of passing urine;
    - vaginal loss and liquor colour should be monitored.

- The partogram is currently recommended for use in established labour by NICE (2014a). However, the authors of a recent Cochrane review (Lavender et al. 2013) stated that they cannot recommend the routine use of partograms for standard labour management and care.

- Recent evidence has highlighted that the spectrum of normal progress in labour may be much wider than previously accepted, particularly up to cervical dilatation of 6 cm (Zhang et al. 2010).

- A vaginal examination is one of many methods of assessment that a midwife can use to monitor the progress of labour (Shepherd and Cheyne 2013); its importance should not be over-emphasised.

- Abdominal palpation, monitoring contractions for frequency, length and strength and observing behavioural cues of the woman are other important midwifery tools. A midwife should use all of her skills to assess labour progress.

- Current NICE guidance (NICE 2014a) states that vaginal examinations should be offered 4-hourly or if there is concern about progress, or in response to a woman's wishes.

- Approximately 20% of women may have the urge to push before full dilatation of the cervix (Charles 2013a). Belief that 'early' pushing will cause an oedematous cervix is based on very little evidence (Perez-Botella and Downe 2006) and instructing a woman at the end of first stage not to push if she has the urge to do so is unnecessary (Charles 2013a).

PROFESSIONAL ACCOUNTABILITY

- It is central to a midwife's role to ensure that, prior to labour onset, women receive good education, particularly about the latent phase of labour. This communication can increase the likelihood of a woman arriving at her chosen birth setting in established labour (RCM 2012d).

- Midwives have an important role in providing the reassurance that women seek – that their experiences during the latent phase of labour are normal (RCM 2012d).

- Midwives should be aware that the care they provide to women during labour can transform their birth experience. Furthermore, poor birth experiences have been shown to be linked to poor perinatal mental health outcomes (RCM 2012a).

- The midwife needs to finely balance the need to assess continually fetal and maternal well-being, to provide adequate, accurate documentation of care provided and to provide ongoing emotional and physical care and support to labouring women.

Further Resources

Royal College of Midwives. *Evidence Based Guidelines for Midwifery-led Care in Labour: Assessing Progress in Labour*,
   https://www.rcm.org.uk/sites/default/files/Assessing%20Progress%20in%20Labour .pdf.

Royal College of Midwives. *Evidence Based Guidelines for Midwifery-led Care in Labour: Latent Phase*,
   https://www.rcm.org.uk/sites/default/files/Latent%20Phase_1.pdf.

Non-pharmacological Analgesia

In general, the aim of non-pharmacological analgesia is to help women cope with pain during labour, as opposed to pharmacological analgesia, which aims to relieve the pain of labour (Jones *et al.* 2012).

In most settings, women would prefer to experience labour without pharmacological pain relief (Downe *et al.* 2015). It is therefore important that practitioners can provide evidence-based information on safe and effective forms of alternative pain relief. In reality, the subject of pain relief in labour is widely discussed and debated within the literature, with much conflicting evidence, due to a range of study types and quality. As such, the Cochrane Pregnancy and Childbirth Group considered the topic deserving of an 'overview of systematic reviews', in order to provide a single document, rather than the many individual Cochrane reviews and countless other studies on the subject (Jones *et al.* 2012).

KEY POINTS

- The use of water for pain relief during labour is not new, with a long history of application in lay and clinical care (Garland 2010).

- Despite some controversy over its use, the most recent Cochrane review found that, for low-risk women, water use in labour reduced the need for epidural analgesia and shortened the first stage of labour, with no adverse effects on the woman or fetus (Cluett and Burns 2012).

- In addition, two recent large observational studies found that the use of water in labour was associated with spontaneous vaginal birth with no adverse effects, particularly for nulliparous women (Burns *et al.* 2012; Henderson *et al.* 2014).

- There is some evidence to suggest that massage, acupuncture and relaxation (yoga, music) may improve labour pain management with few adverse effects (Jones *et al.* 2012).

- Smith *et al.* (2012) found that less pain was reported in women who received massage compared with usual care.

- Acupuncture and acupressure may have a role in reducing pain, increasing satisfaction with pain management and reducing use of pharmacological pain relief (Smith *et al.* 2011a).

- Jones *et al.* (2012) stated that there was insufficient evidence to determine whether TENS (transcutaneous electrical nerve stimulation) should be recommended for use in labour, whereas the individual Cochrane review (Dowswell *et al.* 2009) stated that although evidence is limited, women should have the choice of using TENS in labour. Current NICE guidance (NICE 2014a) advises against its use, yet many women frequently choose this form of pain relief (Bedwell *et al* . 2011).

- The use of self-hypnosis for labour-pain management has been increasing in popularity, despite the most recent Cochrane review showing no conclusive benefit (Madden *et al.* 2012). New evidence from Downe *et al.* (2015) identified that self-hypnosis did not influence epidural use or any other clinical outcomes but it did reduce levels of childbirth fear and anxiety postnatally.
- Smith *et al.* (2011b) were unable to make clinical recommendations either for or against the use of aromatherapy for pain management in labour because of a lack of robust data. However, results from a large observational study suggest that aromatherapy can be effective in reducing maternal anxiety, fear and pain during labour (Burns *et al.* 2000). Some oils are contraindicated in pregnancy (Tiran 2000).

ESSENTIALS OF MIDWIFERY CARE

- There is a clear demand for better quality research with respect to the efficacy and use of non-pharmacological pain relief (Jones *et al.* 2012); however, in the meantime, the midwife should ensure that a woman is provided with the best available evidence to permit informed choice (NMC 2015).
- Low-risk women who choose to labour in water should be supported to do so. Women with risk factors should receive individualised advice. The water temperature should be comfortable for the woman but not above 37.5 °C. The temperatures of the water and the woman should be checked and documented hourly (NICE 2014a).

PROFESSIONAL ACCOUNTABILITY

- Midwives should be committed to supporting a woman's choices for pain relief in labour, regardless of whether this reflects their own values and beliefs (NICE 2014a).
- The midwife must practise within the boundaries of Professional Accountability (RCM 2014). For example, NICE (2014a) states that acupuncture, acupressure and hypnosis should not be offered to women, but also states that midwifery care should support a woman's informed choice.
- Discussions around preferences for pain relief should be fully documented.

Further Resources

Jones, L., Othman, M., Dowswell, T., Alfirevic, Z., Gates, S., Newburn, M., Jordan, S., Lavender, T. and Neilson, J.P. (2012) Pain management for women in labour: an overview of systematic reviews. *Cochrane Database of Systematic Reviews*, Issue 3 (Art. No.: CD009234), doi: 10.1002/14651858.CD009234.pub2, http://onlinelibrary.wiley.com/doi/10.1002/14651858.CD009234.pub2/epdf.

Occipito-posterior Position

Most women will begin labour with their baby in an occipito-anterior (OA) position, often considered to be the optimal position for labour and delivery (Hunter *et al.* 2007). However, in approximately 15–32% of women, the baby will present in the occipito-posterior (OP) position (Simkin 2010). This is more common in nulliparous women.

An OP position has been linked to more painful labour, prolonged labour, obstructed labour and difficult delivery (Hunter *et al.* 2007). However, some authors are keen to emphasise that the OP position is another version of normal and should therefore be treated as such (Reed 2015).

KEY POINTS

- It is important to note that the techniques commonly used to 'diagnose' OP position, such as location of the fetal heart, observing a 'dip' in the maternal belly, Leopold's manoeuvre, vaginal examinations and maternal backache, are not reliable (Simkin 2010; RCM 2012g).

- Ultrasound scans may accurately determine fetal position but the potential risk of repeated use of ultrasound scanning is unknown (Simkin 2010).
- Although 15–32% of women are thought to present with a baby in the OP position, only 5–8% will subsequently give birth to a baby in the OP position (Simkin 2010). The majority of babies therefore will internally rotate to OA.
- Lieberman *et al.* (2005) found that epidural analgesia reduced the likelihood of a fetus internally rotating to OA prior to birth. This may be due to the epidural relaxing the pelvic floor, removing the counter-pressure that enables the fetus to pivot. This may be a contributory factor in the reduction of spontaneous vaginal delivery in women with epidural analgesia.
- OP position during labour has been linked to:
  - prolonged first and second stages of labour;
  - oxytocin augmentation;
  - use of epidural analgesia;
  - chorioamnionitis;
  - assisted vaginal delivery;
  - severe perineal lacerations;
  - caesarean section;
  - excessive blood loss;
  - postpartum infection (Ponkey *et al.* 2003; RCM 2012g).
- There has been some investigation into the antenatal and labour use of specific maternal postures to correct OP positioning. A Cochrane review (Hunter *et al.* 2007) stated that there is no evidence to support the use of a hands-and-knees position antenatally for this purpose. However, it reported that this position does reduce backache during labour and called for further studies to investigate other intrapartum outcomes.

ESSENTIALS OF MIDWIFERY CARE
- A thorough knowledge of physiology and the mechanism of labour is essential.
- Midwives need to be aware that the OP labour may not fit 'traditional' time-scales. Careful, evidence-based explanation of this should be given to women.
- Women should be supported to remain mobile, change position during labour and have access to a birthing pool or bath if desired.
- The birthing environment should lend itself to upright and active labour.
- Continuity of carer should be supported wherever possible.
- It is important to reinforce a woman's belief in her body to birth her baby, including physical and emotional support during a long labour, backache and pain in labour.
- Advice on interventions during labour should be offered with care, without increasing women's feelings of anxiety or predispose her to feelings of failure. Women should be supported in the choices they make (RCM 2012g; Reed 2015).

PROFESSIONAL ACCOUNTABILITY
- Midwives must have competence in a wide range of midwifery skills in order to apply positive actions to support women through an OP labour and birth, along with a sound knowledge of the mechanism of an OP labour (RCM 2012g).

Further Resources

Reed, R. (2015) *In Celebration of the OP Baby*, MidwifeThinking, http://midwifethinking.com/2010/08/13/in-celebration-of-the-op-baby/.

Simkin, P. (2010) The fetal occiput posterior position: state of the science and a new perspective. *Birth*, **37**, 61–71.

Pharmacological Analgesia

The aim of pharmacological analgesia is to relieve the pain of labour (Jones *et al.* 2012). It can usefully be divided into three broad categories: inhaled analgesia; opioid analgesia and regional (epidural) anaesthesia.

Although most women, prior to labour onset, would prefer to labour without the use of pharmacological analgesia (Downe *et al.* 2015), pharmacological analgesia certainly has its place in modern midwifery care. It is important, therefore, that midwives have an understanding of the different types of pharmacological analgesia, including side-effects, to enable and support women to make informed choices (RCM 2012f).

KEY POINTS

- Entonox, a 50:50 mixture of oxygen and nitrous oxide, is currently the most commonly used pharmacological analgesia and NICE (2014a) recommends that it should be available in all birth settings.

- There is some evidence that such inhaled analgesia does effectively relieve pain compared with placebo (Jones *et al.* 2012). It is considered safe for woman and baby but may cause vomiting, nausea and lightheadedness (Jones *et al.* 2012).

- Opioids, including pethidine, meptazinol and diamorphine, are recommended to be available in all birth settings (NICE 2014a). However, their use is somewhat controversial, with concern that much of the effect is sedation and not analgesia (Wee *et al.* 2014), with obvious effects on mobility during labour.

- Ullman *et al.* (2010) stated that although opioids provide limited pain relief in labour, they are associated with adverse effects.

- NICE (2014a) reported these adverse effects as including drowsiness, nausea and vomiting for the woman, and short-term respiratory depression and drowsiness (which may last several days) for her baby. There may also be a negative impact on breastfeeding.

- Maternal satisfaction with opioids as pain relief during labour is 'moderate at best' (Ullman *et al.* 2010).

- There is concern that although it is the most widely used opioid worldwide, pethidine may not be the best option in terms of balancing pain relief with adverse effects. Ullman *et al.* (2010) suggested a need for further quality research. A recent large trial found diamorphine to give superior pain relief but with an associated lengthening of labour (Wee *et al.* 2014).

- Epidural anaesthesia works by blocking sensory nerve impulses as they enter the spinal cord and evidence shows that it effectively manages pain during labour (Jones *et al.* 2012). However, Jones *et al.* (2012) also stated that epidural use leads to more instrumental vaginal births and caesarean sections for fetal distress (although with no difference in the rates of caesarean section overall).

ESSENTIALS OF MIDWIFERY CARE

- It is essential that women make informed choices with respect to the use of pharmacological analgesia and that they are made aware of the risks and benefits (NICE 2014a). Evidence-based information should preferably be given antenatally, but if not it should be discussed during labour, prior to administration (RCM 2012f).

- Women should be able to access pain relief at any point during labour. This may require transfer to an obstetric unit, in which case transfer of care and transfer times should be clearly explained to the woman.
- An anti-emetic should be given alongside opioid administration owing to the risk of nausea and vomiting. Women should be advised not to enter the pool within 2 hours of opioid administration or if they feel drowsy (NICE 2014a).
- Women with epidural anaesthesia are no longer under midwifery-led care; care will be provided in consultation with the obstetric team. NICE (2014a) offer a number of recommendations for the care of women with epidural anaesthesia:
  - Intravenous access should be gained, and a fluid infusion may be required.
  - Hourly checks of the level of sensory block should be carried out.
  - Blood pressure should be monitored every 5 minutes for 15 minutes following epidural establishment and after further boluses.
  - Women should be encouraged to move and adopt comfortable upright positions.
  - Anaesthesia should be continued until after the third stage of labour and perineal repair (if required).
  - Continuous electronic fetal monitoring should be carried out for at least 30 minutes during establishment and further boluses of epidural anaesthesia.
  - Careful monitoring of bladder care will be required owing to the possibility of loss of bladder function. A urinary catheter may be required.

PROFESSIONAL ACCOUNTABILITY

- Midwives should be committed to supporting a woman's choices for pain relief in labour, regardless of whether this reflects their own values and beliefs (NICE 2014a).
- Record keeping is an integral part of a midwife's role (NMC 2009). Discussions around options for pain relief, in addition to administration, should be fully documented.

Further Resources

Jones, L., Othman, M., Dowswell, T., Alfirevic, Z., Gates, S., Newburn, M., Jordan, S., Lavender, T. and Neilson, J.P. (2012) Pain management for women in labour: an overview of systematic reviews. *Cochrane Database of Systematic Reviews*, Issue 3 (Art. No.: CD009234), doi: 10.1002/14651858.CD009234.pub2,
http://onlinelibrary.wiley.com/doi/10.1002/14651858.CD009234.pub2/epdf.

Promoting Normality

Promoting normality is often considered central to a midwife's role during labour and birth (RCM 2015a) although there has been considerable discussion around defining 'normal birth'. The worth of focusing on normal birth has been questioned as it may not be achievable for all women, yet the midwifery care received may transform a woman's birth experience (RCM 2012a). The RCM 'better births' campaign (RCM 2015a) was started in May 2014 in order to focus on normalising birth for all women, including those who may not have a normal birth.

Active Labour and Birth

In developed countries, most women currently labour and give birth lying down (RCM 2012b). Historically, this position may have been promoted by caregivers for ease of practice (Souza *et al.* 2006) before becoming entrenched in Western culture and practice (RCM 2012b).

In cultures not influenced by Western society, women often choose to labour and birth in upright positions (Lawrence *et al.* 2013). This may be physiologically beneficial owing to the force of gravity aiding descent of the fetus, reduced compression on abdominal blood vessels increasing uterine blood flow, thereby aiding contractions, and by giving the woman a sense of control and comfort (Lawrence *et al.* 2013).

KEY POINTS

- Recent Cochrane reviews on maternal position in the first stage of labour (Lawrence *et al.* 2013) and the second stage of labour (Gupta *et al.* 2012) both reported methodological concerns but nonetheless supported the use of upright positions throughout labour and birth.

- The length of the first stage of labour was reduced and there was reduced use of epidural anaesthesia and less likelihood of caesarean section for women who remained upright, compared with recumbent, during first stage (Lawrence *et al.* 2013).

- There was no evidence of increased intervention rates or negative effects on mothers' or babies' well-being (Lawrence *et al.* 2013).

- Gupta *et al.* (2012) reported a reduction in operative delivery and use of episiotomy and fewer abnormal fetal heart rate patterns for women who remained in upright, compared with recumbent, positions during second stage.

- They also found an increased risk of maternal blood loss of more than 500 ml (Gupta *et al.* 2012), although there are methodological concerns surrounding the estimation of blood loss from different maternal positions (RCM 2012b).

- Maternal satisfaction was investigated in both Cochrane reviews but the results were inconclusive.

ESSENTIALS OF MIDWIFERY CARE

- Women should be informed of the benefits and potential risks of upright positions during labour and birth (Gupta *et al.* 2012; Lawrence *et al.* 2013).

- Midwives should be proactive – demonstrating, encouraging and assisting women to assume upright positions during labour and birth (RCM 2012b; NICE 2014a).

- The labour environment should optimise a woman's ability to remain upright and mobile. Furniture and props such as beanbags, mattresses, chairs and birth balls should be available and promoted (RCM 2012b).

- Such support should not be at the cost of listening to a woman's needs; decisions to rest should be supported. There is some evidence that as labour progresses, women show a natural tendency to lie down (Roberts *et al.* 1983)

- Studies by Downe *et al.* (2004) and Roberts *et al.* (2005) were inconclusive on the optimal position for birth if a woman is using epidural anaesthesia; both called for larger studies to be conducted.

PROFESSIONAL ACCOUNTABILITY

- It takes substantial commitment and proactivity from midwives to facilitate upright positions throughout labour and birth, particularly if the labouring woman requires more intensive care, such as the use of continuous electronic fetal monitoring or where intravenous access is required (RCM 2012b).

Further Resources

Royal College of Midwives. *Top Ten Tips for Normality in Birth for Midwives*, https://www.rcm.org.uk/top-ten-tips-for-normality-in-birth-for-midwives.

Environment and Culture

Both the environment (birthplace setting) and the culture (or care model) within which a woman receives her midwifery care can influence mode of birth (Birthplace in England Collaborative Group 2011; Sandall *et al.* 2013) and satisfaction level (Williams *et al.* 2010).

KEY POINTS

- The Maternity Care Working Party (2008) considers a normal birth to be 'without induction, without the use of instruments, not by caesarean section and without general, spinal or epidural anaesthetic before or during delivery'.

- Most women would like to give birth with little or no medical intervention if safe to do so and if they feel able to cope (Maternity Care Working Party 2008).

- Evidence suggests that healthy women with low risk pregnancies should be offered a choice of birthplace setting and be supported in their choice (Birthplace in England Collaborative Group 2011).

- The Birthplace in England Collaborative Group (2011), in their seminal study, found that:
  - Adverse outcomes are uncommon across all birthplace settings but interventions are less common for births planned outside an obstetric unit.
  - For women having their first baby, there is a high chance of transfer to an obstetric unit from other birth settings and there may be a higher risk of an adverse outcome if planning a birth at home.

- Women receiving midwifery-led models of care, compared with other care models, are more likely to experience normal birth parameters and report higher satisfaction levels (Sandall *et al.* 2013).

- Substantial current interest exists in caseload models of midwifery care. For women with uncomplicated pregnancies, caseload models can increase normal birth parameters such as spontaneous vaginal birth (McLachlan *et al.* 2012). Regardless of a woman's 'risk status', they are safe and cost-effective (Tracy *et al.* 2013).

- Caseload models specifically focused on socially disadvantaged women may lead to improved birth outcomes for this group of women (Rayment-Jones *et al.* 2015).

ESSENTIALS OF MIDWIFERY CARE

- All women in labour should receive one-to-one midwifery care (NICE 2014a).

- Owing to lower intervention rates, with no adverse impact on the baby, current NICE guidance (NICE 2014a) states that:
  - Low-risk multiparous women should be advised that birth at home or in a midwifery unit (alongside or freestanding) is particularly suitable for them.

- ○ Low-risk women having their first baby should be advised that birth at a midwifery unit is particularly suitable for them.
- ○ Women with risk factors should receive individualised advice for the most appropriate birth setting for them.
- It is important to remember that midwives are expert professionals skilled in supporting and maximising *normality* regardless of place or type of birth (RCM 2015a).
- Midwives have an important role to play in normalising birth for women who have pre-existing or pregnancy-related conditions (RCM 2015a).

PROFESSIONAL ACCOUNTABILITY
- There should be a culture of compassionate care for each individual woman, recognising the emotionally intense experience of childbirth (NICE 2014a).
- All women should be supported to make a fully informed decision on their choice of birth setting (NICE 2014a).

Further Resources

Royal College of Midwives. *Better Births Initiative*,
    https://www.rcm.org.uk/clinical-practice-and-guidelines/better-births.

National Perinatal Epidemiology Unit (NPEU). *Birthplace in England Research Programme*,
    https://www.npeu.ox.ac.uk/birthplace.

Second Stage of Labour

The second stage of labour is considered to be from full dilatation of the cervix until the birth of the baby. However, the exact point of reaching full dilatation is rarely known. Care during the second stage of labour focuses on continual assessment of fetal and maternal well-being, assessment of fetal descent and rotation and physical and emotional support for the woman. Intervention is not required while maternal and fetal conditions are satisfactory and there is ongoing descent of the presenting part (RCM 2012h). However, if there are any deviations from normal and/or concerns for fetal or maternal well-being, referral to the obstetric team should be implemented in a timely manner. This may include transfer to an obstetric unit.

KEY POINTS

- The care provided by the midwife during the second stage has the potential to transform a woman's experience. Larkin and Begley (2009) suggested that caregivers who are knowledgeable, intuitive and flexible and able to provide individualised care can enhance the labour and birth experience.

- The length of the second stage will be influenced by parity (NICE 2014a), maternal position (Gupta *et al*. 2012), use of epidural anaesthesia (NICE 2014a) and position of the fetus (Simkin 2010).

- Preceding the second stage, there may be a period of 'transition', forming a period of overlap between the first and second stages. During this stage, women can appear increasingly agitated, making distressed requests such as further pain relief after previously coping well, wanting to return home or stating an inability to cope any longer. A noticeable 'rest and be thankful' phase can occur after transition, sometimes termed the passive second stage, characterised by a spacing of contractions before the strong urges to bear down begin, giving a brief chance to rest (Downe and McCourt 2008).

- Evidence suggests that a prolonged second stage increases the risk of postpartum haemorrhage, infection and significant perineal trauma (but with few adverse neonatal outcomes); however, the methodological rigour of several of these studies has been called into question (Altman and Lydon-Rochelle 2006). Rouse *et al*. (2009) suggested that the second stage does not need to be terminated for duration alone.

- Current NICE guidance (NICE 2014a) states that for nulliparous women, the second stage should be completed within 3 hours of the onset of active second stage (2 hours for multiparous women). Transfer to obstetric care, including transfer to an obstetric unit if applicable, is recommended if birth is not imminent after 2 hours (or 1 hour for multiparous women).

ESSENTIAL PHYSIOLOGY

- The characteristics of the second stage include the following:

  - Spontaneous rupture of membranes, if this did not occur in the first stage.

  - A strong urge to push, as a result of powerful, expulsive contractions.

  - Rectal pressure, the feeling of a need to open the bowels; and often a woman will do so.

  - Anal dilation, bulging perineum, vulval gaping, clear descent of the presenting part. Note that some of these will only be visible with certain maternal positions (Chapman and Charles 2013).

- The urge to push is thought to arise from the presenting part stretching the pelvic floor muscles, resulting in a surge of oxytocin release alongside catecholamines, intensifying the positive feedback loop and leading to expulsive contractions. This process is known as the Ferguson reflex (Ferguson 1941).

- As the fetus continues to descend, it must make a number of manoeuvres and rotations in order to pass through the maternal pelvis, down the birth canal and exit (Arya *et al.* 2007).

- These manoeuvres are often termed 'the mechanism of labour'. A sound understanding of the normal *mechanism of labour* should not be underestimated in providing a foundation to recognise deviations from normality. However, it should also be remembered that each labour, woman and fetus are unique.

- In a normal occipito-anterior mechanism, with *descent* comes *increased flexion*. As the head pushes against the pelvic floor, resistance from these muscles causes *internal rotation of the fetal head*, necessary due to the differing dimensions of the maternal pelvis at the brim and the outlet. Once completed, the fetal neck will lie under the pubic arch.

- Epidural anaesthesia may cause a reduction in pelvic floor muscle tone, disrupting the normal mechanism of internal rotation of the fetal head and resulting in malposition (Simkin 2010). This may be a contributory cause of increased instrumental deliveries seen with epidural anaesthesia.

- *Extension of the head* and neck can then occur, leading to the *birth of the head, face and then chin*. This includes *crowning*, which causes an intense stretching and burning sensation as the head passes through the vulval orifice.

- *Restitution* will occur, usually after a short while, to realign the fetal head with the shoulders, which undergo *internal rotation* at this time (Chapman and Charles 2013).

- Although many textbooks state that the anterior shoulder is born first, in many cases the posterior shoulder will be born first (Walsh 2012). This may be influenced by maternal position.

- Malposition of the fetus (occipito-posterior position; see Section 2.1.2) or breech presentation (see Section 4.1) will result in differing mechanisms (Arya *et al.* 2007).

ESSENTIALS OF MIDWIFERY CARE

- As with the first stage of labour, a calm, private, darkened environment should be promoted in order to facilitate oxytocin release (Charles 2013a), ensuring that the positive feedback loop continues.

- Verbal reassurance is often a key part of second-stage care but should be delivered calmly and usually quietly. Charles (2013a) outlined the key midwifery skill of balancing the need for a verbal injection of energy as encouragement for the woman, without this becoming a 'cacophony of shouting and exhorting'.

- Alongside an ongoing assessment of the colour of liquor, NICE (2014a) states that the following maternal observations should be recorded and documented:
  - half-hourly documentation of contraction frequency;
  - hourly blood pressure;
  - 4-hourly temperature;
  - frequency of passing urine.

- The midwife should observe and monitor uterine contractions, ongoing descent and rotation of the fetus and fetal and maternal well-being in order to be satisfied that the second stage of labour is continuing normally.

- There is no need to carry out a vaginal examination to confirm full dilatation of the cervix, although this is commonly done. However, NICE (2014a) recommends that a vaginal examination should be offered hourly during the second stage or in response to a woman's wishes.

- Throughout the second stage, the fetal heart should be ascultated after a contraction for at least 1 minute, at least every 5 minutes. The maternal pulse should be palpated every 15 minutes to differentiate between the two (NICE 2014a).
- Ongoing consideration should be given to the woman's position, hydration, coping strategies and pain relief throughout the second stage.
- Upright and active birth positions should be encouraged (Gupta *et al.* 2012). Midwives should be proactive; enabling women to assume upright positions during the second stage (RCM 2012b; NICE 2014a).
- Women should be enabled to push spontaneously, without direction; and only when they have the urge to do so.
- Directed pushing or Valsalva pushing, where a woman is instructed to take and hold her breath and push as long and hard as she can, is not necessary. Although resulting in a shorter second stage, it also leads to a decrease in urodynamic factors (Prins *et al.* 2011).
- If an epidural is *in situ*, the woman may not feel contractions building and a certain amount of direction may be indicated. Switching off the epidural prior to commencing pushing can be distressing for the woman and does not increase the spontaneous birth rate (Torvaldsen *et al.* 2004).
- Controlled birth of the fetal head has been shown to reduce the likelihood of perineal trauma (Albers and Borders 2007). NICE (2014a) supports either a hands-on or hands-poised approach to birth of the fetal head.
- It is important then to wait for restitution before the birth of the body, unless this follows spontaneously.
- Carroli and Mignini (2009), in a Cochrane review, concluded that restrictive episiotomy policies appear to have a number of benefits compared with policies based on routine episiotomy. NICE (2014a) states that episiotomies should not be carried out routinely. However, the procedure may be indicated on occasion, for example to expedite the birth of a compromised fetus.
- Delayed cord clamping and immediate skin-to-skin contact should be supported (NICE 2014a). There is no need to remove the baby from the mother for routine observations such as weighing and recording initial temperature (NICE 2014a). APGAR scores should be recorded at 1 and 5 minutes, along with the length of time to establish regular respirations.

PROFESSIONAL ACCOUNTABILITY

- A midwife must show competence in their understanding of the normal physiology and mechanisms of labour in order to support, using positive actions, women who may have a malpositioned fetus (RCM 2012g).
- Midwives must also recognise when a deviation from normality has occurred and referral to the wider multidisciplinary team is required.
- Record keeping is an integral part of a midwife's role (NMC 2009) and the timely documentation of care provided is an essential part of second-stage care.

Further Resources

Royal College of Midwives. *Evidence Based Guidelines for Midwifery-led Care in Labour: Second Stage of Labour*,
  https://www.rcm.org.uk/sites/default/files/Second%20Stage%20of%20Labour.pdf.

Pilu, G. Animation of the mechanism of the second stage of labour,
  https://www.youtube.com/watch?v=b2h4ERLpn0w.

Perineal Trauma

Approximately 85% of women will sustain some form of perineal trauma during childbirth (Smith *et al.* 2013), although the severity of this can vary considerably. Perineal trauma is described in terms of the degree of tear sustained. A first-degree tear comprises injury to the perineal skin only, a second-degree comprises injury to the perineal muscles, a third-degree tear involves the anal sphincter complex (and is further subdivided depending on the extent) and a fourth-degree tear involves the anal sphincter complex and anal epithelium (Abbott *et al.* 2010). Third- and fourth-degree tears together are often classified as 'obstetric anal sphincter injuries' (OASIS) and, although relatively rare (~1–3% of women), there is particular concern attributed to this type of perineal trauma in childbirth due to its association with significant short- and long-term maternal morbidity (Smith *et al.* 2013).

KEY POINTS

- There is considerable discussion in the literature around potential causes of perineal trauma, particularly OASIS, and whether any of these causes are preventable. There are three particular areas of current focus:
  - method of pushing;
  - position of the practitioner's hands at delivery ('hands-on' or 'hands-off');
  - the use of specific techniques (e.g. digital perineal stretching, warm compress) to reduce trauma.
- The significance of directed pushing for perineal trauma remains unclear. Aasheim *et al.* (2011) stated that the pushing technique has no influence, whereas Smith *et al.* (2013) found that directed pushing may have had some influence on the likelihood of OASIS occurrence.
- The position of the hands at delivery has attracted considerable attention since the publication of the HOOP trial (McCandlish *et al.* 1998). However, the Cochrane review by Aasheim *et al.* (2011) found no effect of hand position on OASIS occurrence but did find that the hands-poised technique reduced the incidence of episiotomy.
- Digital perineal stretching or massage during the second stage does not reduce or increase the likelihood of perineal trauma (Aasheim *et al.* 2011; Smith *et al.* 2013). However, evidence suggests that antenatal perineal massage from 35 weeks' gestation decreases the incidence of perineal trauma and therefore women should be given information on how to massage effectively (Beckmann and Stock 2013).
- Application of a warm compress has been shown to reduce the incidence of OASIS (Aasheim *et al.* 2011).

ESSENTIALS OF MIDWIFERY CARE

- Smith *et al.* (2013) found that planning birth in hospital, as opposed to a freestanding midwifery unit or at home, led to an increased risk of perineal trauma.
- Current NICE guidance (NICE 2014a) reflects the findings of the recent Cochrane review, stating that either a hands-on or a hands-poised technique may be used to facilitate spontaneous birth. Maternal choice for a warm compress should be supported.
- After the birth, the perineum should be inspected for trauma using an aseptic technique as soon as is practicable. Shortly after the completion of the third stage of labour is often a suitable moment for woman and midwife. If required, suturing should be carried out in a timely manner, using a technique such as PEARLS[1]; which has been shown to improve evidence-based practice (Ismail *et al.* 2013).
- If OASIS is suspected, timely confirmation and repair by an obstetrician should follow. This may require transfer to an obstetric unit.

---

[1] Perineal assessment and repair longitudinal study.

- The woman should be informed of any perineal trauma obtained and any suturing required. In addition, the midwife should discuss postnatal perineal care (see Section 3.3) with the woman, including the signs and symptoms of infection (NICE 2014b).

PROFESSIONAL ACCOUNTABILITY

- Competence is required in perineal trauma assessment and repair. However, recent research suggests that few midwives are currently using evidence-based suturing methods to repair perineal trauma. In addition, midwives overall do not feel confident in their ability to assess or repair perineal trauma all of the time (Bick et al. 2012). Recognising limitations and seeking appropriate assistance when required are therefore important.

- Once competence is gained, midwives have a duty to maintain their skills and keep up-to-date with new techniques and research evidence (NMC 2015).

- Record keeping is an integral part of a midwife's role (NMC 2009) and should be completed for all perineal trauma. This may require the use of incidence forms for OASIS.

Further Resources

Royal College of Midwives. *RCM i-learn: MaternityPEARLS – Perineal Repair and Suturing*, http://www.ilearn.rcm.org.uk/course/info.php?id=11.

Waterbirth

There is some evidence that using water for labour is beneficial for low-risk women, with few ill-effects for the woman or newborn (Cluett and Burns 2012). The picture is less clear for giving birth in water, mainly owing to a paucity of quality research on the subject. The difficulty of conducting rigorous research into waterbirth is widely recognised (Charles 2013b). The body of evidence surrounding waterbirth is growing, however, and it is a popular choice for women. Midwives should be able to give evidence-based information with respect to this birthing method.

KEY POINTS

- Cluett and Burns (2012) found no evidence of increased adverse effects to the woman or newborn from waterbirth; although this was based on just three trials and the authors call for further research.

- Burns et al. (2012) found that for women who used a pool during labour, most had a spontaneous birth (88.9%) and 58.3% had a waterbirth.

- Women's experiences of waterbirth appear to be positive (Nutter et al. 2014) and associated with greater birth satisfaction (Cluett and Burns 2012), although this finding was from just one trial.

- NICE (2014a) guidance states that women should be informed that 'there is insufficient high-quality evidence either to support or to discourage giving birth in water'.

- Upright positions should be supported during the second stage (Gupta et al. 2012). There is some evidence that waterbirth promotes the use of more physiological, and more upright, birthing positions (Henderson et al. 2014).

- The issue of perineal trauma and waterbirth remains controversial; however, there are questions about the rigour of some of the studies and therefore further quality research is warranted:
  - Cluett and Burns (2012) found no difference in perineal trauma between women who had a waterbirth and those who birthed on land.
  - Otigbah et al. (2000) reported fewer instances of perineal trauma with waterbirth; Cortes et al. (2011) identified an increase in severe perineal trauma.

○ Henderson *et al.* (2014) found a reduction in the use of episiotomy, with a corresponding increase in second-degree tears, for women who gave birth in water.

- Both Burns *et al.* (2012) and Henderson *et al.* (2014) cautioned against undue traction on the cord owing to the possibility of cord snap. Burns *et al.* (2012) reported 20 incidences of cord snap in a large British observational study, 18 of which occurred during waterbirth.

- Burns *et al.* (2012) found that planned place of birth influences outcomes for pool use; for example, more nulliparous women in community settings, compared with hospital settings, had a spontaneous birth. This is particularly relevant as most of the research conducted to date has been in obstetric units, whereas pool use is common practice in community settings.

ESSENTIALS OF MIDWIFERY CARE

- Women should be supported to make an informed choice with respect to giving birth in water.

- The temperatures of the water and the woman should be checked and documented hourly (NICE 2014a). The water temperature should not be above 37.5 °C.

- Midwives should have access to training in the use of water for labour and birth, and protocols should be in place to support practice (RCM 2012i).

- Although cited by some as a concern during waterbirth, there is no evidence to support an increased risk of infection to woman or baby. However, pools should be thoroughly cleaned between uses, following the manufacturer's guidelines (NICE 2014a).

- Charles (2013b) gave a detailed account of midwifery care during waterbirth, a summary of which is offered below to aid revision:

  ○ As with a land-based second stage, keep the room darkened, quiet and private.
  ○ Carry out second-stage observations according to current NICE guidance (NICE 2014a).
  ○ There is usually no need to observe the perineum. If indicated, and if the woman consents, an easy-to-clean or disposable mirror can be used.
  ○ Adopt a hands-off approach to the birth, due to an unconfirmed risk that touching the fetal head could cause a premature gasp from the baby.
  ○ Once visible, ensure that the fetal head remains under water until complete birth of the baby. If the woman does raise herself out of the water, encourage her to remain standing, although she does not need to exit the pool.
  ○ There should be no need to assist with the delivery and the woman can bring the baby to the surface herself if she wishes.
  ○ Babies born into water may not cry and may not breathe instantly. This is rarely cause for concern. If need be, the baby can be briefly lifted up into the cool air to stimulate the first breath. Support delayed cord clamping and immediate skin-to-skin contact.

PROFESSIONAL ACCOUNTABILITY

- Providing midwifery care to support birth in water should be considered a core midwifery competence (Charles 2013b).

- Midwives should have access to training in the use of water for labour and birth and protocols should be in place to support practice (RCM 2012i).

Further Resources

Charles, C. (2013) Water for labour and birth, in *The Midwife's Labour and Birth Handbook*, 3rd edn (eds V. Chapman and C. Charles), John Wiley & Sons, Chichester, pp. 117–129.

Third Stage of Labour

This is defined as the period from the birth of the baby until complete expulsion of the placenta and membranes (Begley *et al.* 2011). This is an important stage of the childbirth process and the one perhaps most eagerly anticipated by the woman and her birth partner; however, their needs and expectations can frequently be overlooked where routine tasks dominate the birth room. The third stage of labour has often been recognised as the most hazardous stage of labour because of the risk of severe bleeding and, for many women around the world, it remains a significant risk. In the United Kingdom, 11 women died from haemorrhage in the triennium 2010–2012: the third most common cause of direct maternal death (Knight *et al.* 2014). The low rate of maternal mortality associated with the third stage of labour is attributed to a widespread policy of active management (Harris 2011).

KEY POINTS NICE (2014a) advises that:

- Active management of the third stage of labour should be recommended to women because it is associated with a lower risk of postpartum haemorrhage.
- If low-risk women choose physiological management, they should be supported in their choice.
- During pregnancy, the benefits and risks of physiological and active management should be clearly explained to women in easily understandable terms, thereby facilitating informed choice.
- *Active management* of the third stage of labour:
  - shortens the third stage compared with physiological management;
  - is associated with nausea and vomiting (N and V) for around 100/1000 women;
  - is associated with around a 13/1000 risk of haemorrhage of more than 1 litre;
  - is associated with around a 14/1000 risk of a blood transfusion.
- *Physiological management* of the third stage of labour:
  - is associated with N and V for around 50/1000 women;
  - is associated with around a 29/1000 risk of haemorrhage of more than 1 litre;
  - is associated with around a 40/1000 risk of a blood transfusion.
- The component of an active management care package that reduces bleeding remains unknown (Fahy *et al.* (2010).

ESSENTIAL PHYSIOLOGY

- The placenta usually begins to separate from the uterine wall with the contraction that delivers the baby's body.
- Further contraction and retraction of uterus greatly reduce the surface area of the myometrium. This predominantly accounts for separation of the placenta because:
  - Maternal blood in the intervillous spaces is forced back into the veins of the decidua but cannot return to the maternal circulation because of the contracted and retracted state of the uterus.
  - The congested veins therefore rupture and the blood loss shears off the villi from the decidua, thereby separating the placenta.
  - The greatly reduced surface area within the uterus means that the placenta, being inelastic, is shorn off the decidua and rests in the lower uterine segment.
- A small gush of blood appears per vagina that indicates placental separation. Signs of descent are lengthening of the cord and a raised, globular fundus that can be easily palpated abdominally.
- The placenta usually appears at the vulva fetal side first, with the membranes trailing behind and blood loss neatly contained within (Schultze method). If it descends on its

side, it will appear maternal side first (Matthews Duncan method) and more blood loss is visible, hence the nickname 'dirty' Duncan.

- Bleeding from the torn blood vessels within the large placental site must be rapidly controlled in order to prevent catastrophic haemorrhage; at term, approximately 500 ml/min is exchanged between the feto-maternal system:
  - The unique, uterine spiral muscle fibres interweave the torn blood vessels, forming 'living ligatures' and control blood loss.
  - The uterine walls appose, enhancing the contracted uterus and forming a natural compress.
  - There is a transient rise in maternal clotting factors.
  - A fibrin mesh rapidly forms over the placental site.
- The placental site heals by exfoliation and does not leave a scar (Blackburn 2013; Harris 2011).

ACTIVE MANAGEMENT
Begley et al. (2011) identified that active management:

- Reduces the risk of severe bleeding (>1000 ml).
- Increases maternal blood pressure.
- Is associated with vomiting, afterpains and re-admission to hospital with bleeding.
- Reduces babies' birthweight.

Key principles:

- Administration of an oxytocic drug with birth of the anterior shoulder. NICE (2014a) currently advises the use of oxytocin as it is associated with fewer side-effects than oxytocin with ergometrine; however, this is dependent on local guidelines.
- Early clamping and cutting of the cord. NICE (2014a) advises that this should be performed after 1 minute and before 5 minutes. Delaying cord clamping may benefit the baby by increasing blood volume but more research is needed to be sure (Begley et al. 2011).
- Placenta and membranes are delivered by controlled cord traction.

PHYSIOLOGICAL OR EXPECTANT MANAGEMENT
- Is associated with reduced bleeding (Fahy et al. 2010).
- For low-risk women, a physiological third stage may pose no greater risk of excessive blood loss (Giacalone et al. 2000; Dixon et al. 2013).

Key principles:

- No oxytocic drug is administered.
- The cord is clamped once it has stopped pulsating or following delivery of the placenta and membranes.
- The placenta and membranes are delivered by maternal effort, usually aided by gravity and the promotion of oxytocin release, e.g. an undisturbed, ambient birth environment; breastfeeding.

ESSENTIALS OF MIDWIFERY CARE
- Promote attachment and bonding by facilitating time and privacy for the new family, including skin-to-skin contact. A key influencing factor is to delay non-essential tasks.
- Observation of maternal pulse, well-being and vaginal bleeding throughout the third stage of labour is an essential component of midwifery care.

- Promotion of an ambient birth environment is especially important for physiological management, e.g. warmth, dimly lit room, privacy, skin-to-skin contact, breastfeeding.

- Recognition of the signs of placental separation and descent.

- Diagnosis of a prolonged third stage of labour: 30 minutes for active management and 60 minutes for physiological management.

- Advise a change from physiological to active management where:
  o haemorrhage occurs;
  o the placenta is not delivered within 1 hour of birth.

- Thorough inspection of placenta and membranes to establish if complete and to exclude abnormalities.

- Estimation of measured blood loss.

- Prompt collection of cord/maternal blood if Rh negative.

- Prompt perineal repair if indicated using an evidence-based technique, for example, MaternityPEARLS (see Section 2.3.1) (Harris 2011; NICE 2014a).

PROFESSIONAL ACCOUNTABILITY

- Midwives have a professional duty to maintain competent clinical skills in order to facilitate and respect maternal choice. This includes familiarity with current best evidence and local guidelines.

- The provision of timely information is important in order to facilitate informed choice.

- Contemporaneous record keeping in clear plans of care is required.

Further Resources

Royal College of Midwives. *Evidence Based Guidelines for Midwifery-led Care in Labour: Third Stage of Labour,*
https://www.rcm.org.uk/sites/default/files/Third%20Stage%20of%20Labour.pdf.

Challenges

Cord Prolapse

This is defined as the descent of the umbilical cord through the cervix either alongside (occult) or in front of (overt) the presenting part where there are ruptured membranes. Cord presentation occurs when the umbilical cord lies between the presenting part and the cervix, in the presence or absence of intact membranes (RCOG 2014).

KEY POINTS

- Cord prolapse is an obstetric emergency and is associated with a high perinatal mortality rate, which the RCOG (2014) reported as around 91/1000 births.

- The incidence of cord prolapse is 0.1–0.6% and higher with a breech presentation at just over 1%.

- It is associated with multiple pregnancies, prematurity and congenital malformations.

- Fetal asphyxia is caused by cord compression and umbilical arterial vasospasm that may result in encephalopathy and cerebral palsy.

- The core principles of managing a cord prolapse are to alleviate cord compression and expedite the birth (RCOG 2014).

MANAGEMENT AND CARE The RCOG Green top Guideline No. 50, *Umbilical Cord Prolapse*, provides comprehensive and evidence-based guidance (RCOG 2014), a summary of which is offered below to aid revision:

- *Alleviate cord compression:*
  - Elevate the presenting part either manually or by filling the bladder.
  - Assist the woman to adopt the knee–chest or exaggerated Sims position (left lateral position with her head down and left hip raised on a pillow). The latter is advised if transferring the woman by ambulance.

- *Deliver the baby:*
  - Caesarean section is recommended if vaginal birth is not imminent.
  - Vaginal birth can be attempted if the cervix is fully dilated and the delivery can be accomplished easily and speedily. This may be particularly relevant for a multiparous woman.

- Women and their partners should have an opportunity to discuss the event shortly after birth and ask questions. The midwife may also value a debriefing session with his/her supervisor of midwives.

- Community midwives are recommended to carry a Foley catheter as part of their obstetric emergency kit.

- Accurate and contemporaneous record keeping is of critical importance during an obstetric emergency, especially if transfer from the community to hospital is required.

PROCESSIONAL ACCOUNTABILITY

- Midwives must maintain their skills and competence with the recognition and management of obstetric emergencies, for example, regular participation in 'skills drills'. This may be particularly important for those working in freestanding midwifery units or attending homebirths.

- Opportunities to practise skills with other members of the multiprofessional team are desirable in order to maximise smooth transition of care, for example, community midwives working alongside paramedics.

- Effective communication is essential during any obstetric emergency.

Eclampsia

Eclampsia is the occurrence of seizures where there is pre-eclampsia and is thought to occur where there is severe cerebral vasospasm, haemorrhage, ischaemia or oedema (Gilbert 2011). However, despite its association with pre-eclampsia, in up to 20% of cases a woman may present with eclamptic convulsions prior to any signs or symptoms of pre-eclampsia (Sibai 2005). Eclampsia is a significant cause of maternal mortality, particularly in the developing world where it is the third most common cause of death (WHO 2015). In the United Kingdom, however, deaths from pre-eclampsia and eclampsia, including HELLP syndrome and acute fatty liver of pregnancy, are at their lowest recorded levels (Knight et al. 2009). This is attributed to the introduction of magnesium sulfate for the treatment of eclampsia, together with clear quality standards from NICE.

KEY POINTS
- The underlying cause of eclampsia is still not fully understood (Duley et al. 2010).
- It is difficult to predict who is at risk of eclampsia, as only 1–2% of women with severe pre-eclampsia will go on to develop the condition. However, certain risk factors for developing eclampsia have been identified from several studies:
  - pre-existing hypertension;
  - low (under 20 years) and high (35 or more years) maternal age;
  - nulliparity;
  - low socio-economic status;
  - pre-pregnancy obesity and excessive weight gain during pregnancy;
  - extended birth interval and pre-existing hypertension (Coghill et al. 2011).
- Eclampsia follows from severe pre-eclampsia, defined by NICE (2010) as severe hypertension and proteinuria or mild or moderate hypertension and proteinuria with one or more of the following signs:
  - severe headache;
  - visual disturbances, such as blurring or flashing lights;
  - severe pain just below the ribs or vomiting;
  - papilloedema[2];
  - signs of clonus[3];
  - liver tenderness;
  - HELLP syndrome;
  - platelet count falling to below 100×10^9/litre.
  - abnormal liver enzymes (ALT or AST rising to above 70 IU/l).
- During an eclamptic seizure, convulsions usually begin with facial twitching, followed by generalized rigidity of muscles, then coma. Respirations cease during convulsions because of muscle spasms but will resume following the convulsion (Gilbert 2011).
- Be alert to the 30% of eclampsia cases that occur during the postnatal period (Sibai 2005).
- Eclampsia can be very alarming for the woman and her family and therefore sensitive psychological support should be offered (Boyle and McDonald, 2011).

MANAGEMENT AND CARE
The following are adapted from NICE (2010) and Gilbert (2011):

---

[2] Swelling of the optic disc caused by raised intracranial pressure.
[3] Involuntary, rhythmic muscular spasms.

- Regular antenatal care ensures assessment of pregnant women for clinical signs of pre-eclampsia, the aim being to detect the condition early and thus prevent the onset of serious complications such as eclampsia.

- Hypertensive disease in pregnancy complicated by pre-eclampsia/eclampsia requires regular antenatal care, early recognition and referral, appropriate treatment and timely delivery (Ghulmiyyah and Sibai 2012).

- Prior to the onset of a convulsion, women may experience certain symptoms such as headache, epigastric pain, blurred vision, nausea and vomiting, confusion or irritability (Briley 2013). However, there may be no warning at all.

- Immediate actions during and/or following a convulsion should be as follows (Briley 2013):
  - Keep calm and *summon help*. Do not leave the woman alone.
  - Use the **ABC** (airway, breathing, circulation) approach.
  - *Ensure that the woman is safe*; remove dangerous objects; do not restrain or place anything in her mouth.
  - Once the convulsion has finished, place the woman in left-lateral and give *facial oxygen* if available to increase utero-placental blood flow.
  - Note the time and duration of the convulsion.

- After these initial actions:
  - Take a full set of *observations*, including pulse oximetry if available.
  - Gain *intravenous access*.
  - Catheterise.
  - *Continuously monitor BP and fluid balance*.
  - Monitor the fetus using electronic fetal monitoring if possible (expecting poor fetal condition immediately after the fit).
  - Both the woman and her birth partners will need reassurance. Speaking in calm tones throughout the convulsion and afterwards may help (Briley 2013).

- Maintain a quiet environment.

- *Administer IV magnesium sulfate* to women with severe hypertension who have, or have previously had, an eclamptic fit, in accordance with the Collaborative Eclampsia Trial regime (The Eclampsia Trial Collaborative Group 1995):
  - A loading dose of 4 g should be given IV over 5 minutes.
  - An infusion of 1 g/hour should then be maintained for 24 hours.
  - Recurrent seizures should be treated with a further dose of 2–4 g over 5 minutes.
  - Maternal toxicity is rare when therapeutic levels are carefully monitored.

- *Administer antihypertensive drugs* such as labetalol, hydralazine or nifedipine.

- Respiration rate and pulse oximetry should be recorded at least hourly, and bloods monitored to ensure that magnesium levels remain within the therapeutic range.

- Observe the woman carefully for uterine contractions as seizures frequently stimulate labour.

- Base labour and birth decision on the woman's preference and clinical condition – the only cure is ending the pregnancy.

PROFESSIONAL ACCOUNTABILITY

- Midwives must respond calmly and appropriately to emergency situations, including those where a woman has sudden onset of eclampsia.

- As with all aspects of midwifery, good documentation is an essential requirement of good and effective practice.

Further Resources

Action on Pre-eclampsia, http://action-on-pre-eclampsia.org.uk/.

Primary Postpartum Haemorrhage

A woman is considered to have suffered a primary postpartum haemorrhage (PPH) if there is loss of 500 ml or more of blood from the genital tract within 24 hours of the birth of a baby (RCOG 2011). Primary PPH can be classified as minor (500–1000 ml without signs or symptoms of shock) or major (more than 1000 ml, or less than this but with clinical signs or symptoms of shock) (RCOG 2011).

Primary PPH is an important cause of maternal morbidity and mortality (Giacalone *et al.* 2000; Sheldon *et al.* 2013). It is therefore critically important that midwives can recognise and act upon primary PPH when it does occur.

KEY POINTS

- Worldwide, PPH is the main cause of maternal mortality (Nour 2008), while in the United Kingdom it accounts for approximately 10% of all maternal deaths attributed to obstetric causes (Knight *et al.* 2014).

- Both internationally and in the United Kingdom, the incidence of PPH in high-income countries is rising (Knight *et al.* 2009). In England its recorded incidence nearly doubled from 7% of all births in 2004–2005 to 13% in 2011–2012 (Knight *et al.* 2014).

- Many 'risk factors', which increase the risk of a woman having a PPH, have been suggested, with varying levels of research evidence. These include, but are not limited to:
  - method of third-stage management;
  - obstetric interventions;
  - first pregnancy;
  - maternal obesity;
  - macrosomic baby;
  - multiple pregnancy;
  - prolonged or augmented labour;
  - chorioamnionitis;
  - pre-eclampsia;
  - maternal anaemia;
  - antepartum haemorrhage (Mousa *et al.* 2014).

- Although often cited, high multiparity does not appear to be a risk factor (Mousa *et al.* 2014).

- Although many risk factors have been identified, PPH can often occur unexpectedly in low-risk women (Mousa *et al.* 2014).

- NICE guidance (NICE 2014a) recommends that all women should be advised to have active management of the third stage of labour to reduce the risk of haemorrhage. However, there is debate within the literature whether for low-risk women a physiological third stage may pose no greater risk of excessive blood loss (Giacalone *et al.* 2000; Dixon *et al.* 2013).

- NICE guidance (NICE 2014a) also states, 'If a woman at low risk of postpartum haemorrhage requests physiological management of the third stage, support her in her choice'. Such women should be advised to change from physiological to active management if there is concern about the level of blood loss or if the placenta remains *in situ* after 1 hour (NICE 2014a).

MANAGEMENT AND CARE

- Women with risk factors for PPH should be advised to give birth in an obstetric unit.

- Once a PPH has been identified, the midwife needs to instigate simultaneously several components of management (RCOG 2011; NICE 2014a):

○ *Call for help.* For a minor PPH, this may be an obstetrician, anaesthetist and senior midwife. For a major PPH, it should include senior midwives, senior obstetricians and senior anaesthetists; in addition to communication with haematologists, the blood transfusion laboratory and porters. Communication with the woman and her birth partner is equally important.

○ *Initiate prompt clinical treatment:*

  – Insertion of an indwelling catheter.
  – Uterine massage.
  – Uterotonic drugs.
  – Intravenous fluids.
  – Controlled cord traction (if the placenta is not delivered).

○ *Continually assess blood loss and maternal condition:*

  – Obtain intravenous access at two sites.
  – Carry out an ABC (airway, breathing, circulation) approach to resuscitation.
  – Lie the woman flat and keep her warm.
  – Commence oxygen and intravenous fluids (use up to 2 l of warmed crystalloid fluid until blood is available).
  – Organise the administration of blood products.

○ *Identify the cause and stop the bleeding as soon as possible.* Bleeding from a PPH relates to one of the 'four Ts':

  – *Tone* (a lack of uterine tone, the most common cause of PPH).
  – *Trauma* (usually severe perineal but may be high vaginal or cervical tears).
  – *Tissue* (retained products in the uterus).
  – *Thrombin* (abnormality of clotting factors).

○ Do not hesitate to commence *bimanual compression* once the four Ts have been assessed and persistent bleeding continues.

○ *Ongoing monitoring and investigation:*

  – Obtain bloods for FBC; group and save; clotting.
  – Commence maternal observations every 5 minutes (blood pressure, pulse and respiration rate) and temperature every 15 minutes. Ensure accurate documentation of all observations.

• If the PPH occurs in a community setting, the priority is to transfer the woman to an obstetric unit as a matter of urgency, alongside implementing the procedures above. Bimanual compression to stem bleeding may be required until arrival at an obstetric unit and/or bleeding is stemmed.

PROFESSIONAL ACCOUNTABILITY

• Effective communication between clinical staff is essential, particularly in situations that require prompt decision-making and action, such as postpartum haemorrhage (Knight *et al.* 2014).

• The use of a structured communication tool such as SBAR (Situation, Background, Assessment, Recommendation) may be very useful and effective in such situations (Knight *et al.* 2014).

• The midwife must remain vigilant within the scope of her role, remaining attentive to maternal observations and condition, escalating abnormal observations and recognising a deteriorating woman (Knight *et al.* 2014).

• Accurate documentation is crucial. A scribe should be allocated in any PPH situation. They should maintain a record of observations, fluid balance, blood, blood products and all procedures carried out (RCOG 2011).

Further Resources

RCOG (2011) *Postpartum Haemorrhage, Prevention and Management*, Green-top Guideline No. 52, Royal College of Obstetricians and Gynaecologists, London, https://www.rcog.org.uk/en/guidelines-research-services/guidelines/gtg52/.

Shoulder Dystocia

Shoulder dystocia is an obstetric emergency and all midwives must be able to recognise it and respond appropriately. It usually occurs when the anterior fetal shoulder impacts on the maternal symphysis pubis. Less commonly, it can occur when the posterior shoulder impacts on the sacral promontory (RCOG 2012).

KEY POINTS

- There can be significant perinatal morbidity and mortality associated with shoulder dystocia, even when managed appropriately. There is increased maternal risk of PPH and OASIS. Post-traumatic stress disorder and postnatal depression may occur (Miskelly 2013).

- Fetal risk includes brachial plexus injury, occurring in 2–16% of shoulder dystocia incidents (RCOG 2012). Although most cases resolve without permanent injury, it is the most common cause of litigation related to shoulder dystocia cases (RCOG 2012). Other fetal complications include fractured clavicle, hypoxia, bruising, tissue damage and, in severe cases, fetal death (Miskelly 2013).

- Although many risk factors for shoulder dystocia have been identified, most occur without any identified risk. Therefore, clinicians should be aware of existing risk factors in labouring women, but should always be alert to the possibility of shoulder dystocia even in their absence (RCOG 2012).

- Pre-labour risk factors include a previous shoulder dystocia, suspected macrosomia (fetal weight estimated to be >4.5 kg), diabetes mellitus and maternal body mass index >30 kg/m^2. Intrapartum risk factors include a prolonged first stage, prolonged second stage, oxytocin augmentation, induction of labour and assisted vaginal birth (RCOG 2012).

- Induction of labour at term can reduce the incidence of shoulder dystocia in women with gestational diabetes (RCOG 2012).

- A previous shoulder dystocia does not require subsequent routine elective caesarean section, but factors such as the severity of any previous neonatal or maternal injury, predicted fetal size and maternal choice should all be considered and discussed with the woman (RCOG 2012).

MANAGEMENT AND CARE

- Shoulder dystocia is often preceded by a slow delivery of the fetal head and often 'turtle-necking' will be seen, where the head retracts back against the perineum. However, shoulder dystocia should only be diagnosed when the body does not deliver during the next contraction, when gentle traction is applied (RCOG 2012).

- It is important that shoulder dystocia is not over-diagnosed (Miskelly 2013).

- Once a shoulder dystocia has been diagnosed, further traction should be avoided (RCOG 2012).

- The RCOG (2012) offers comprehensive guidelines, a summary of which is provided below to aid revision:

  ○ Shoulder dystocia should be managed systematically. A scribe should be appointed.

  ○ *Call for help* immediately after recognition of shoulder dystocia. This may require urgent transfer to an obstetric unit. State clearly that 'this is shoulder dystocia' to the obstetric team.

  ○ *Maternal pushing should be discouraged* and fundal pressure should not be used.

  ○ The *McRoberts manoeuvre* widens the planes of the pelvis and is a simple, rapid and effective intervention that should be performed first. *Suprapubic pressure* should be used to improve the effectiveness of the McRoberts manoeuvre.

○ An episiotomy is not always necessary but may be required to give access for manoeuvres.

○ Internal manoeuvres or *'all-fours' position* should be used if the McRoberts manoeuvre and suprapubic pressure fail. For a mobile woman without epidural anaesthesia and a single midwife, the all-fours position may be more appropriate initially. The alternative method should then be used if necessary.

○ For internal manoeuvres, the woman should be brought to the end of the bed.

○ A hand should be inserted posteriorly and an attempt made to *remove the posterior fetal arm*. This will reduce the diameter of the shoulders by the width of the arm,

○ Alternatively, *internal manoeuvres* to rotate the shoulders may be performed first:

  – Applying pressure on the posterior aspect of the posterior shoulder adducts the shoulders, thereby reducing their diameter.
  – If that fails, an attempt should be made to apply pressure on the posterior aspect of the anterior shoulder to adduct the shoulders and encourage rotation into the oblique diameter of the pelvis.

○ These procedures should be repeated systematically until further help arrives.

• The woman and birth partners may wish to debrief with a healthcare professional soon after the birth and/or again at a later date. However, evidence on the efficacy of postnatal debriefing is inconsistent. Some evidence suggests that it is beneficial if used specifically when requested by women (Meades *et al.* 2011). However, NICE (2014b) does not recommend the use of a formal debrief.

PROFESSIONAL ACCOUNTABILITY

• A midwife will require courage when faced with shoulder dystocia in order to stay calm and carry out the appropriate procedures in a timely fashion.

• Documentation is critically important. Neonatal brachial plexus injury, the majority of which occurs during shoulder dystocia, is the third most litigated obstetric-related complication in the UK (RCOG 2012). Good practice and good documentation of such events help to reduce litigation (Miskelly 2013).

Further Resources

RCOG (2012) *Shoulder Dystocia*, Green-top Guideline No. 42, 2nd edn, Royal College of Obstetricians and Gynaecologists, London,
    https://www.rcog.org.uk/globalassets/documents/guidelines/gtg42_25112013.pdf.

References

Aasheim, V., Nilsen, A.B.V., Lukasse, M. and Reinar, L.M. (2011) Perineal techniques during the second stage of labour for reducing perineal trauma. *Cochrane Database of Systematic Reviews*, Issue 12 (Art. No.: CD006672), doi: 10.1002/14651858.CD006672.pub2.

Abbott, D., Atere-Roberts, N., Williams, A., Oteng-Ntim, E. and Chappell, L.C. (2010) Obstetric anal sphincter injury. *BMJ*, **341**, c3414.

Albers, L.L. and Borders, N. (2007) Minimizing genital tract trauma and related pain following spontaneous vaginal birth. *Journal of Midwifery and Womens Health*, **52**, 246–253.

Altman, M.R. and Lydon-Rochelle, M.T. (2006) Prolonged second stage of labor and risk of adverse maternal and perinatal outcomes: a systematic review. *Birth*, **33** (4), 315–322.

Arya, R., Whitworth, M. and Johnston, T.A. (2007) Mechanism and management of normal labour. *Obstetrics, Gynaecology and Reproductive Medicine*, **17** (8), 227–231.

Bailit, J.L., Dierker, L., Blanchard, M.H. and Mercer, B.M. (2005) Outcomes of women presenting in active versus latent phases of spontaneous labour. *British Journal of Obstetrics and Gynaecology*, **105** (1), 77–79.

Beckmann, M.M. and Stock, O.M. (2013) Antenatal perineal massage for reducing perineal trauma. *Cochrane Database of Systematic Reviews*, Issue 4 (Art. No.: CD005123), doi: 10.1002/14651858.CD005123.pub3.

Bedwell, C., Dowswell, T., Neilson, J. and Lavender, T. (2011) The use of transcutaneous electrical nerve stimulation (TENS) for pain relief in labour: a review of the evidence. *Midwifery*, **27**, e141–e148.

Begley, C.M., Gyte, G.M.L., Murphy, D.J., Devane, D., McDonald, S.J. and McGuire, W. (2011) Active versus expectant management for women in the third stage of labour. *Cochrane Database of Systematic Reviews*, Issue 11 (Art. No.: CD007412), doi: 10.1002/14651858.CD007412.pub3.

Bick, D.E., Ismail, K.M.K., Macdonald, S., Thomas, P., Tohill, S. and Kettle, C. (2012) How good are we at implementing evidence to support the management of birth related perineal trauma? A UK wide survey of midwifery practice. *BMC Pregnancy and Childbirth*, **12**, 57.

Birthplace in England Collaborative Group (2011) Perinatal and maternal outcomes by planned place of birth for healthy women with low risk pregnancies: the Birthplace in England National Prospective Cohort Study. *BMJ*, **343**, d7400.

Blackburn, S.T. (2013) *Maternal, Fetal, and Neonatal Physiology: a Clinical Perspective*, 4th edn, Elsevier Saunders, Maryland Heights, MO.

Boyle, M. and McDonald, S. (2011) Pre-eclampsia and eclampsia, in *Emergencies Around Childbirth: a Handbook for Midwives*, 2nd edn (ed. M. Boyle), Radcliffe Publishing, London, pp. 55–69.

Briley, A. (2013) Preeclampsia, in *The Midwife's Labour and Birth Handbook*, 3rd edn (eds V. Chapman and C. Charles), John Wiley & Sons, Chichester, pp. 318–335.

Burns, E., Blamey, C., Ersser, S.J., Lloyd, A.J. and Barnetson, L. (2000) The use of aromatherapy in intrapartum midwifery practice: an observational study. *Complementary Therapies in Nursing and Midwifery*, **6** (1), 33–34.

Burns, E., Boulton, M.G., Cluett, E., Cornelius, V.R. and Smith, L.A. (2012) Characteristics, Interventions, and outcomes of women who used a birthing pool: a prospective observational study. *Birth*, **39** (3), 192–202.

Carroli, G. and Mignini, L. (2009) Episiotomy for vaginal birth. *Cochrane Database of Systematic Reviews*, Issue 1 (Art. No.: CD000081), doi: 10.1002/14651858.CD000081.pub2.

Chapman, V. and Charles, C. (eds) (2013) *The Midwife's Labour and Birth Handbook*, 3rd edn, John Wiley & Sons, Chichester.

Charles, C. (2013a) Labour and normal birth, in *The Midwife's Labour and Birth Handbook*, 3rd edn (eds V. Chapman and C. Charles), John Wiley & Sons, Chichester, pp. 1–38.

Charles, C. (2013b) Water for labour and birth, in *The Midwife's Labour and Birth Handbook*, 3rd edn (eds V. Chapman and C. Charles), John Wiley & Sons, Chichester, pp. 117–129.

Cluett, E.R. and Burns, E. (2012) Immersion in water in labour and birth. *Cochrane Database of Systematic Reviews*, Issue 2 (Art. No.: CD000111), doi: 10.1002/14651858.CD000111.pub3.

Coghill, A.E., Hansen, S. and Littman, A.J. (2011) Risk factors for eclampsia: a population-based study in Washington State, 1987–2007. *American Journal of Obstetrics and Gynecology*, **205** (6), 553.e1–553.e7.

Cortes, E., Basra, R. and Kelleher, C.J. (2011) Waterbirth and pelvic floor injury: a retrospective study and postal survey using ICIQ modular long form questionnaires. *European Journal of Obstetrics and Gynecology and Reproductive Biology*, **155**, 27–30.

Dixon, L., Tracey, S.K., Guilliland, K., Fletcher, L., Hendry, C. and Pairman, S. (2013) Outcomes of physiological and active third stage labour care amongst women in New Zealand. *Midwifery*, **29**, 67–74.

Downe, S. and McCourt, C. (2008) From being to becoming: reconstructing childbirth knowledges, in *Normal Childbirth: Evidence and Debate*, 2nd edn (ed. S. Downe), Churchill Livingstone Elsevier, Edinburgh, pp. 3–24.

Downe, S., Gerrett, D. and Renfrew, M.J. (2004) A prospective randomised trial on the effect of position in the passive second stage of labour on birth outcome in nulliparous women using epidural analgesia. *Midwifery*, **20**, 157–168.

Downe, S., Finlayson, K., Melvin, C., Spiby, H., Ali, S., Diggle, P., Gyte, G., Hinder, S., Miller, V., Slade, P., Trepel, D., Weeks, A., Whorwell, P. and Williamson, M. (2015) Self-hypnosis for intrapartum pain management in pregnant nulliparous women: a randomised controlled trial of clinical effectiveness. *British Journal of Obstetrics and Gynaecology*, **122**, 1226–1234.

Dowswell, T., Bedwell, C., Lavender, T. and Neilson, J.P. (2009) Transcutaneous electrical nerve stimulation (TENS) for pain management in labour. *Cochrane Database of Systematic Reviews*, Issue 2 (Art. No.: CD007214), doi: 10.1002/14651858.CD007214.pub2.

Duley, L., Gülmezoglu, A.M., Henderson-Smart, D.J. and Chou, D. (2010) Magnesium sulphate and other anticonvulsants for women with pre-eclampsia. *Cochrane Database of Systematic Reviews*, Issue 11 (Art. No.: CD000025), doi: 10.1002/14651858.CD000025.pub2.

Fahy, K., Hastie, C., Bisits, A., Marsh, C., Smith, L. and Saxton, A. (2010) Holistic physiological care compared with active management of the third stage of labour for women at low risk of postpartum haemorrhage: a cohort study. *Women and Birth*, **23** (4), 146–152.

Ferguson, J.K.W. (1941) A study of the motility of the intact uterus at term. *Surgery, Gynecology and Obstetrics*, **73**, 359–366.

Garland, D. (2010) *Revisiting Waterbirth: an Attitude to Care*, Palgrave Macmillan, Basingstoke.

Ghulmiyyah, L. and Sibai, B.M. (2012) Maternal mortality from preeclampsia/eclampsia. *Seminars in Perinatology*, **36**, 56–59.

Giacalone, P.L., Vignal, J., Daures, J.P., Boulot, P., Hedon, B. and Laffargue, F. (2000) A randomised evaluation of two techniques of management of the third stage of labour in women at low risk of postpartum haemorrhage. *British Journal of Obstetrics and Gynaecology*, **107**, 396–400.

Gilbert, E. (2011) *Manual of High Risk Pregnancy and Delivery*, Mosby, St Louis, MO.

Gupta, J.K., Hofmeyr, G.J. and Shehmar, M. (2012) Position in the second stage of labour for women without epidural anaesthesia. *Cochrane Database of Systematic Reviews*, Issue 5 (Art. No.: CD002006), doi: 10.1002/14651858.CD002006.pub3.

Harris, T. (2011) Care in the third stage of labour, in *Mayes' Midwifery*, 14th edn (eds S. Macdonald and J. Magill-Cuerden), Baillière Tindall Elsevier, Edinburgh, pp. 535–548.

Henderson, J., Burns, E.E., Regalia, A.L., Casarico, G., Boulton, M.G. and Smith, L.A. (2014) Labouring women who used a birthing pool in obstetric units in Italy: prospective observational study. *BMC Pregnancy and Childbirth*, **14**, 17.

Hodnett, E.D., Gates, S., Hofmeyr, G.J., Sakala, C. and Weston, J. (2011) Continuous support for women during childbirth. *Cochrane Database of Systematic Reviews*, Issue 2 (Art. No.: CD003766), doi: 10.1002/14651858.CD003766.pub3.

Hunter, S., Hofmeyr, G.J. and Kulier, R. (2007) Hands and knees posture in late pregnancy or labour for fetal malposition (lateral or posterior). *Cochrane Database of Systematic Reviews*, Issue 4 (Art. No.: CD001063), doi: 10.1002/14651858.CD001063.pub3.

Ismail, K.M.K., Kettle, C., Macdonald, S.E., Tohill, S., Thomas, P.W. and Bick, D. (2013) Perineal Assessment and Repair Longitudinal Study (PEARLS): a matched-pair cluster randomized trial. *BMC Medicine*, **2013**, 11, 209.

Jones, L., Othman, M., Dowswell, T., Alfirevic, Z., Gates, S., Newburn, M., Jordan, S., Lavender, T. and Neilson, J.P. (2012) Pain management for women in labour: an overview of systematic reviews. *Cochrane Database of Systematic Reviews*, Issue 3 (Art. No.: CD009234), doi: 10.1002/14651858.CD009234.pub2.

Kamel, R.M. (2010) The onset of human parturition. *Archives of Gynecology and Obstetrics*, **281**, 975–982.

Knight, M., Callaghan, W.M., Berg, C., Alexander, S., Bouvier-Colle, M.-H., Ford, J.B., Joseph, K.S., Lewis, G., Liston, R.M., Roberts, C.L., Oats, J. and Walker, J. (2009) Trends in postpartum hemorrhage in high resource countries: a review and recommendations from the International Postpartum Hemorrhage Collaborative Group. *BMC Pregnancy and Childbirth*, **9**, 55.

Knight, M., Kenyon, S., Brocklehurst, P., Neilson, J., Shakespeare, J. and Kurinczuk, J.J. (eds), on behalf of MBRRACE-UK (2014) *Saving Lives, Improving Mothers' Care – Lessons Learned to Inform Future Maternity Care from the UK and Ireland Confidential Enquiries into Maternal Deaths and Morbidity 2009–2012*, National Perinatal Epidemiology Unit, University of Oxford, Oxford.

Larkin, P. and Begley, C.M. (2009) Women's experiences of labour and birth: an evolutionary concept analysis. *Midwifery*, **25** (2), e49–e59.

Lavender, T., Hart, A. and Smyth, R.M.D. (2013) Effect of partogram use on outcomes for women in spontaneous labour at term. *Cochrane Database of Systematic Reviews*, Issue 7 (Art. No.: CD005461), doi: 10.1002/14651858.CD005461.pub4.

Lawrence, A., Lewis, L., Hofmeyr, G.J. and Styles, C. (2013) Maternal positions and mobility during first stage labour. *Cochrane Database of Systematic Reviews*, Issue 10 (Art. No.: CD003934), doi: 10.1002/14651858.CD003934.pub4.

Lieberman, E., Davidson, K., Lee-Parritz, A. and Shearer, E. (2005) Changes in fetal position during labor and their association with epidural analgesia. *Obstetrics and Gynecology*, **105**, 974–982.

Madden, K., Middleton, P., Cyna, A.M., Matthewson, M. and Jones, L. (2012) Hypnosis for pain management during labour and childbirth. *Cochrane Database of Systematic Reviews*, Issue 11 (Art. No.: CD009356), doi: 10.1002/14651858.CD009356.pub2.

Maternity Care Working Party (2008) *Making Normal Birth a Reality: Consensus Statement from the Maternity Care Working Party*, NCT/RCM/RCOG, London.

McCandlish, R., Bowler, U., van Asten, H., Berridge, G., Winter, C., Sames, L., Garcia, J., Renfrew, M. and Elbourne, D. (1998) A randomised controlled trial of care of the perineum during second stage of normal labour. *British Journal of Obstetrics and Gynaecology*, **105**, 1262–1272.

McLachlan, H.L., Forster, D.A., Davey, M.A., Farrell, T., Gold, L., Biro, M.A., Albers, L., Flood, M., Oats, J. and Waldenstromh, U. (2012) Effects of continuity of care by a primary midwife (caseload midwifery) on caesarean section rates in women of low obstetric risk: the COSMOS randomised controlled trial. *British Journal of Obstetrics and Gynaecology*, **119**, 1483–1492.

Meades, R., Pond, C., Ayer, S, and Warren, F. (2011) Postnatal debriefing: have we thrown the baby out with the bathwater? *Behaviour Research and Therapy*, **49**, 367–372.

Miskelly, S. (2013) Emergencies in labour and birth, in *The Midwife's Labour and Birth Handbook*, 3rd edn (eds V. Chapman and C. Charles), John Wiley & Sons, Chichester, pp. 271–291.

Mousa, H.A., Blum, J., Abou El Senoun, G., Shakur, H. and Alfirevic, Z. (2014) Treatment for primary postpartum haemorrhage. *Cochrane Database of Systematic Reviews*, Issue 2 (Art. No.: CD003249), doi: 10.1002/14651858.CD003249.pub3.

NICE (2008) *Inducing Labour*, NICE Clinical Guideline CG70, National Institute for Health and Clinical Excellence, London.

NICE (2010) *Hypertension in Pregnancy: the Management of Hypertensive Disorders During Pregnancy*, NICE Clinical Guideline CG107, National Institute for Health and Clinical Excellence, London.

NICE (2014a) *Intrapartum Care for Healthy Women and Babies*, NICE Clinical Guideline CG190, National Institute for Health and Care Excellence, London.

NICE (2014b) *Postnatal Care Up to 8 Weeks After Birth*, NICE Clinical Guideline CG37, National Institute for Health and Care Excellence, London.

NMC (2009) *Record Keeping: Guidance for Nurses and Midwives*, Nursing and Midwifery Council, London.

NMC (2015) *The Code: Professional Standards of Practice and Behaviour for Nurses and Midwives*, Nursing and Midwifery Council, London.

Nour, N.M. (2008) An introduction to maternal mortality. *Reviews in Obstetrics and Gynecology*, **1** (2), 77–81.

Nutter, E., Meyer, S., Shaw-Battista, J. and Marowitz, A. (2014) Waterbirth: an integrative analysis of peer-reviewed literature. *Journal of Midwifery and Women's Health*, **59**, 286–319.

Otigbah, C., Dhanjal, M.K., Harsworth, G. and Chard, T. (2000) A retrospective comparison of water births and conventional vaginal deliveries. *European Journal of Obstetrics and Gynecology and Reproductive Biology*, **91**, 15–20.

Perez-Botella, M. and Downe, S. (2006) Stories as evidence: the premature urge to push. *British Journal of Midwifery*, **14** (11), 636–642.

Ponkey, S.E., Cohen, A.P., Heffner, L.J. and Lieberman, E. (2003) Persistent fetal occiput posterior position: obstetric outcomes. *Obstetrics and Gynecology*, **101**, 915–920.

Prins, M., Boxem, J., Lucas, C. and Hutton, E. (2011) Effect of spontaneous pushing versus Valsalva pushing in the second stage of labour on mother and fetus: a systematic review of randomised trials. *British Journal of Obstetrics and Gynaecology*, **118**, 662–670.

Rayment-Jones, H., Murrells, T. and Sandall, J. (2015) An investigation of the relationship between the caseload model of midwifery for socially disadvantaged women and childbirth outcomes using routine data – a retrospective, observational study. *Midwifery*, **31**, 409–417.

RCM (2012a) *Evidence Based Guidelines for Midwifery-led Care in Labour: Supporting Women in Labour*, Royal College of Midwives, London.

RCM (2012b) *Evidence Based Guidelines for Midwifery-led Care in Labour: Positions for Labour and Birth*, Royal College of Midwives, London.

RCM (2012c) *Evidence Based Guidelines for Midwifery-led Care in Labour: Assessing Progress in Labour*, Royal College of Midwives, London

RCM (2012d) *Evidence Based Guidelines for Midwifery-led Care in Labour: Latent Phase*, Royal College of Midwives, London

RCM (2012e) *Evidence Based Guidelines for Midwifery-led Care in Labour: Supporting and Involving Women's Birth Companions*, Royal College of Midwives, London.

RCM (2012f) *Evidence Based Guidelines for Midwifery-led Care in Labour: Understanding Pharmacological Pain Relief*, Royal College of Midwives, London.

RCM (2012g) *Evidence Based Guidelines for Midwifery-led Care in Labour: Persistent Lateral and Posterior Fetal Positions at the Onset of Labour*, Royal College of Midwives, London.

RCM (2012h) *Evidence Based Guidelines for Midwifery-led Care in Labour: Second Stage of Labour*, Royal College of Midwives, London.

RCM (2012i) *Evidence Based Guidelines for Midwifery-led Care in Labour: Immersion in Water for Labour and Birth*, Royal College of Midwives, London.

RCM (2014) *Position Statement: Complementary Therapies and Natural Remedies*, Royal College of Midwives, London.

RCM (2015a) *Better Births Initiative*, Royal College of Midwives, London, https://www.rcm.org.uk/clinical-practice-and-guidelines/better-births (accessed 4 August 2015).

RCM (2015b) *Rupturing Membranes*, Royal College of Midwives, London, http://www.rcmnormalbirth.org.uk/rupturing-membranes/ (acessed 6 August 2015).

RCOG (2011) *Postpartum Haemorrhage, Prevention and Management*, Green-top Guideline No. 52, Royal College of Obstetricians and Gynaecologists, London, https://www.rcog.org.uk/en/guidelines-research-services/guidelines/gtg52/ (accessed 24 November 2015).

RCOG (2012) *Shoulder Dystocia*, Green-top Guideline No. 42, 2nd edn, Royal College of Obstetricians and Gynaecologists, London, https://www.rcog.org.uk/globalassets/documents/guidelines/gtg42_25112013.pdf (accessed 23 November 2015).

RCOG (2014) *Umbilical Cord Prolapse*, Green-top Guideline No. 50, Royal College of Obstetricians and Gynaecologists, London, https://www.rcog.org.uk/globalassets/documents/guidelines/gtg-50-umbilicalcordprolapse-2014.pdf (accessed June 2015).

Reed, R. (2015) *In Celebration of the OP Baby*, MidwifeThinking, http://midwifethinking.com/2010/08/13/in-celebration-of-the-op-baby/ (accessed 26 September 2015).

Roberts, C.L., Algert, C.S., Cameron, C.A. and Torvaldsen, S. (2005) A meta-analysis of upright positions in the second stage to reduce instrumental deliveries in women with epidural analgesia. *Acta Obstetrica et Gynecologica Scandinavica*, **84**, 794–798.

Roberts, J.E., Mendez-Bauer, C. and Wodell, D.A. (1983) The effects of maternal position on uterine contractility and efficiency. *Birth*, **10**, 243–249.

Rouse, D.J., Weiner, S.J., Bloom, S.L., Varner, M.W., Spong, C.Y., Ramin, S.M., Caritis, S.N., Peaceman, A.M., Sorokin, Y., Sciscione, A., Carpenter, M.W., Mercer, B.M., Thorp, J.M., Malone, F.D., Harper, M., Iams, J.D. and Anderson, G.D., for the Eunice Kennedy Shriver National Institute of Child Health and Human Development Maternal–Fetal Medicine Units Network (2009) Second-stage labor duration in nulliparous women: relationship to maternal and perinatal outcomes. *American Journal of Obstetrics and Gynecology*, **201**, 357.e1–357.e7.

Sandall, J., Soltani, H., Gates, S., Shennan, A. and Devane, D. (2013) Midwife-led continuity models versus othermodels of care for childbearing women. *Cochrane Database of Systematic Reviews*, Issue 8 (Art. No.: CD004667), doi: 10.1002/14651858.CD004667.pub3.

Sheldon, W.R., Durocher, J., Winikoff, B., Blum, J. and Trussell, J. (2013) How effective are the components of active management of the third stage of labour? *BMC Pregnancy and Childbirth*, **13**, 46.

Shepherd, A. and Cheyne, H. (2013) The frequency and reasons for vaginal examinations in labour. *Women and Birth*, **26**, 49–54.

Sibai, B. (2005) Diagnosis, prevention and management of eclampsia. *Journal of Obstetrics and Gynaecology*, **105** (2), 402–410.

Simkin, P. (2010) The fetal occiput position: state of the science and a new perspective. *Birth*, **37** (1), 61–71.

Smith, C.A., Collins, C.T., Crowther, C.A. and Levett, K.M. (2011a) Acupuncture or acupressure for pain management in labour. *Cochrane Database of Systematic Reviews*, Issue 7 (Art. No.: CD009232), doi: 10.1002/14651858.CD009232.

Smith, C.A., Collins, C.T. and Crowther, C.A. (2011b) Aromatherapy for pain management in labour. *Cochrane Database of Systematic Reviews*, Issue 7 (Art. No.: CD009215), doi: 10.1002/14651858.CD009215.

Smith, C.A., Levett, K.M., Collins, C.T. and Jones, L. (2012) Massage, reflexology and other manual methods for pain management in labour. *Cochrane Database of Systematic Reviews*, Issue 2 (Art. No.: CD009290), doi: 10.1002/14651858.CD009290.pub2.

Smith, L.A., Price, N., Simonite, V. and Burns, E.E. (2013) Incidence of and risk factors for perineal trauma: a prospective observational study. *BMC Pregnancy and Childbirth* **13**: 59.

Souza, J.P., Miquelutti, M.A., Cecatti, J.G. and Makuch, M.Y. (2006) Maternal position during the first stage of labor: a systematic review. *Reproductive Health*, **3**, 10.

The Eclampsia Trial Collaborative Group (1995) Which anticonvulsant for women with eclampsia? Evidence from the Collaborative Eclampsia Trial. *The Lancet*, **345**, 1455–1463.

Tiran, D. (2000) *Clinical Aromatherapy for Pregnancy and Childbirth*, 2nd edn. Edinburgh: Churchill Livingstone.

Torvaldsen, S., Roberts, C.L., Bell, J.C. and Raynes-Greenow, C.H. (2004) Discontinuation of epidural analgesia late in labour for reducing the adverse delivery outcomes associated with epidural analgesia. *Cochrane Database of Systematic Reviews*, Issue 4 (Art. No.:CD004457), doi: 10.1002/14651858.CD004457.pub2.

Tracy, S.K., Hartz, D.L., Tracy, M.B., Allen, J., Forti, A., Hall, B., White, J., Lainchbury, A., Stapleton, H., Beckmann, M., Bisits, A., Homer, C., Foureur, M., Welsh, A. and Kildea, S. (2013) Caseload midwifery care versus standard maternity care for women of any risk: M@NGO, a randomised controlled trial. *The Lancet*, **382**, 1723–1732.

Ullman, R., Smith, L.A., Burns, E., Mori, R. and Dowswell, T. (2010) Parenteral opioids for maternal pain management in labour. *Cochrane Database of Systematic Reviews*, Issue 9 (Art. No.: CD007396), doi: 10.1002/14651858.CD007396.pub2.

Walsh, D. (2011) Care in the first stage of labour, in *Mayes' Midwifery*, 14th edn (eds S. Macdonald and J. Magill-Cuerden), Baillière Tindall Elsevier, Edinburgh, pp. 483–508.

Walsh, D. (2012) *Evidence and Skills for Normal Labour and Birth: a Guide for Midwives*, 2nd edn, Routledge, Abingdon.

Wee, M.Y.K., Tuckey, J.P., Thomas, P.W. and Burnard, S. (2014). A comparison of intramuscular diamorphine and intramuscular pethidine for labour analgesia: a two-centre randomised blinded controlled trial. *BJOG*, **121**, 447–456.

Westbury, B. (2015) The power of environment. *The Practising Midwife*, **18** (6), 24–26.

Williams, K., Lago, L., Lainchbury, A. and Eager, K. (2010) Mothers' views of caseload midwifery and the value of continuity of care at an Australian regional hospital. *Midwifery*, **26**, 615–621.

WHO (2015) *Maternal Mortality*, Fact Sheet No. 348, World Health Organization, Geneva.

Zhang, J., Landy, H.J., Branch, W., Burkman, R., Herman, S., Gregory, K.D., Hatjis, C.G., Ramirez, M.M., Bailit, J.L., Gonzalez-Quintero, V.H., Hibbard, J.U., Hoffman, M.K., Kominiarek, M., Learman, L.A., Veldhuisen, P.V., Toendle, J. and Reddy, U.M., for the consortium on Safe Labor (2010) Contemporary patterns of spontaneous labor with normal neonatal outcomes. *Obstetrics and Gynecology*, **116** (6), 1281–1287.

PART III

Postnatal Care

Contraception and Sexual Health

Women will generally spend more of their reproductive lifetime preventing pregnancy than experiencing it. The choice of contraceptive methods can be confusing for women; however, the right choice is important if a reasonable gap between pregnancies is the desired outcome. Given that ovulation can resume as early as 28 days following childbirth (FSRH 2009), midwives have a clear role in the provision of up-to-date contraceptive health advice to women, including the availability of emergency contraception.

Short and long-term sexual health morbidities as a result of childbirth are both common and distressing for women. Midwives are ideally placed to recognise the impact of perineal trauma and initiate targeted interventions to support women's recovery and promote optimal sexual health.

KEY POINTS The FSRH (2009) offers extensive guidelines for postnatal sexual health, a summary of which is offered below to aid revision:

- Contraception is not required for 21 days postpartum, based on the earliest ovulation for non-breastfeeding women being 28 days and sperm surviving in the genital tract for up to 7 days.
- Women who are breastfeeding and wish to avoid pregnancy should be advised to use contraception. However, they should be informed that the lactational amenorrhoea method is over 98% effective in preventing pregnancy if:
  - they are less than 6 months postpartum;
  - amenorrhoeic;
  - fully breastfeeding.
- The progestogen only pill (POP) can be started at any time postpartum by both breastfeeding and non-breastfeeding women.
- Combined hormonal contraception (CHC) should not be started within the first 3 weeks postpartum because of the risk of thrombosis. Women who are breastfeeding should avoid CHC during the first 6 weeks as the evidence to support its use safely is unclear.
- The benefits of long-acting reversible contraception should be highlighted to all postpartum women.
- Progestogen-only injectable methods can be started at any time postpartum for non-breastfeeding women. Implants can usually be inserted at 21–28 days postpartum and can be used for both breastfeeding and non-breastfeeding women.
- Emergency hormonal contraception can be used by breastfeeding and non-breastfeeding women after 21 days, or an emergency copper intrauterine device after 28 days.
- Perineal trauma (see Section 2.3.1) during childbirth is a frequent occurrence and has significant effects on women's sexual health:
  - Psychological (Priddis *et al.* 2014), for example, avoidance of sexual intimacy.
  - Reduced libido; reduced vaginal lubrication (Rathfisch *et al.* 2010).
- Anal sphincter injury accounts for around 18% of all vaginal births (Farrar *et al.* 2014). Sequelae include perineal pain, dyspareunia, defaecatory dysfunction and urinary and faecal incontinence.

ESSENTIALS OF MIDWIFERY CARE
- Midwives are ideally placed to create opportunities for women and their partners to discuss sexual health issues, for example, when advising women about perineal wound care and/or contraception. NICE (2006) recommends that this discussion takes place within 2–6 weeks following birth and that the midwife (or other healthcare professional) initiates referral if indicated.

- Midwives should discuss methods of contraception during the antenatal and postnatal period (FSRH 2009) and, as a minimum, during the first postpartum week (NICE 2006).
- Regardless of the choice of contraception, midwives should encourage the use of condoms as these can be used without restriction during the puerperium and will prevent the transmission of most sexually acquired infections (FSRH 2009).
- NICE (2006) advises that:
  - Women should be asked about resumption of sexual intercourse and possible dyspareunia 2–6 weeks after the birth and, if anxiety about resuming intercourse is expressed, this should be sensitively explored.
  - Women with perineal trauma who experience dyspareunia should be offered an assessment of the perineum.
  - Water-based lubricant gel can be advised to ease discomfort during intercourse.
- The FSRH (2009) advises that women and their partners can be reassured by the following:
  - The time to resume sexual activity will vary between couples and there is no recommended time frame, other than both partners needing to be physically and emotionally ready.
  - Sexual desire or sex drive may be low in the first few months.
  - Any difficulties or concerns should be discussed with a healthcare professional.

PROFESSIONAL ACCOUNTABILITY
- Under Article 42 of the EU Midwifery Directive, midwives have a responsibility in the *provision of sound family planning information and advice'*.
- Do not underestimate women's anxiety about resumption of sexual intercourse following childbirth or sexual health problems. Women should be encouraged to discuss any concerns with sensitivity and compassion.

Further Resources

Faculty of Sexual and Reproductive Healthcare, http://www.fsrh.org/.

Facilitating Breastfeeding

The support of breastfeeding women remains a central tenet of skilled midwifery care. The advantages to the baby are well known and firmly established as part of antenatal breastfeeding education. However, the health benefits to women are also significant and should therefore be equally celebrated and promoted to women and their families.

Breastfeeding conveys a number of significant health advantages for mother and baby. For example, it is associated with significant reductions in the rate of infant gastrointestinal and respiratory illness (Duijts *et al.* 2010). For women, breastfeeding reduces the risk of breast cancer and is one of the key protective strategies identified by the World Cancer Research Fund (World Cancer Research Fund/American Institute for Cancer Research 2010). There are clear links between breastfeeding and reductions in childhood obesity (Harder *et al.* 2005) and maternal type 2 diabetes (Liu *et al.* 2010).

When women intend to breastfeed but are subsequently unable to do so, they deserve the same level of midwifery care and support. This is particularly important given the emerging links between breastfeeding intentions, subsequent infant feeding choice and risk of postnatal depression (Borra *et al.* 2015). Breastfeeding is therefore an important public health concern that extends beyond infant feeding issues.

KEY POINTS

- Exclusive breastfeeding is recommended for the first 6 months of an infant's life (WHO 2011).
- The most recent (and the last one to be conducted) infant feeding survey (McAndrew *et al.* 2012) identified the following:
  - The initial breastfeeding rate was 81%.
  - This rate fell to 69% at 1 week, 55% at 6 weeks and 34% at 6 months.
  - The highest rates of breastfeeding were in older mothers; women from minority ethnic groups and women with increased socio-economic markers, for example, professional background.
- All maternity care providers should implement an externally evaluated and structured programme that promotes breastfeeding, using the UNICEF Baby Friendly Initiative (BFI) as a minimum standard (NICE 2006).
- The number of maternity units achieving UNICEF Baby Friendly accreditation tripled between 2001 and 2010 (UNICEF 2010).
- More than one-quarter of women report that they would have liked more help with feeding their babies (Redshaw and Henderson 2015).
- The BFI (2010) identified the key reasons for women stopping breastfeeding as:
  - sore and painful breasts;
  - anxiety that their baby is not getting enough milk;
  - inability to attach their baby successfully.

ESSENTIAL PHYSIOLOGY

- During pregnancy, progesterone and oestradiol antagonise high circulating volumes of prolactin to prevent milk production.
- The process whereby lactation is initiated is known as *lactogenesis*.
- Following birth, levels of progesterone and oestrogen fall; levels of prolactin and oxytocin rise.
- Prolactin is released by the anterior pituitary gland and is responsible for milk production. Oxytocin, released by the posterior pituitary gland, stimulates contraction of the myoepithelial cells in the breast and milk is then propelled along the lactiferous duct to the ampulla.

- A neurohormonal reflex known as the 'let down' reflex acts on prolactin and oxytocin and is stimulated by the infant suckling at the breast. The reflex can also be triggered by the sight, smell, sound or touch of the baby.

- Milk ejection involves both neural and hormonal response. Tactile receptors for both oxytocin and prolactin are located in the nipple, hence tactile stimulation is the most important trigger for the milk ejection reflex.

- Prolactin is released on a supply and demand principle. When the baby stops suckling, prolactin inhibiting factor is released by the hypothalamus and milk production stops.

- *Galactopoiesis* is the establishment of a mature milk supply when major changes in milk composition occur.

- It is dependent on an effective and maintained hypothalamic–pituitary axis and frequent breastfeeding. (Lawrence and Lawrence 1999; Ackerman 2011; Blackburn 2013).

ESSENTIALS OF MIDWIFERY CARE WHO/UNICEF (1989) first identified the 10 steps that help facilitate successful breastfeeding in a joint statement:

- A written breastfeeding policy that is routinely communicated to all staff involved in the support of breastfeeding women.

- Relevant staff to receive training in the required skills to implement the policy.

- Informing all pregnant women about the benefits and management of breastfeeding.

- Helping new mothers initiate breastfeeding within 30 minutes of giving birth.

- Demonstrating how to breastfeed and maintain lactation, even where the mother is separated from her baby.

- Not giving any food or drink to the newborn, other than breast milk (unless medically indicated).

- Practising consistent rooming-in to allow mothers and babies to stay together at all times.

- Encouraging breastfeeding on demand.

- Not offering pacifiers to breastfeeding infants.

- Facilitating breastfeeding support groups and referring women to them on discharge from hospital.

In addition, the NICE (2006) quality standards for postnatal care and the BFI (2010) breastfeeding care pathway include specific guidelines for starting and continuing breastfeeding. A summary of both to aid revision is provided below.

Starting successful breastfeeding:

- Provide women with culturally appropriate *information* about the benefits of breastfeeding, the benefits of colostrum and the timing of the first breastfeed within the first day following birth.

- The *support* that women receive in the first few days following birth can significantly influence their confidence and perseverance with breastfeeding.

- Avoid separating the woman and her baby during the first hour following birth for routine procedures.

- Facilitate women to have *skin-to-skin contact* with their babies as soon as possible after the birth and then enquire about proposed method of feeding.

- Offer skilled breastfeeding support (not necessarily from a midwife) to permit comfortable *positioning of the mother* and *correct attachment of the baby*. Additional support may be required for some women, for example, those who are recovering from caesarean section.

Continuing successful breastfeeding:

- Advise women that healthy babies generally stop feeding when they are satisfied and should be offered the second breast only if they do not appear to be satisfied following a feed from one breast.

- Reassure women that brief discomfort at the start of a breastfeed in the first few days is not uncommon but should not persist. Sore or cracked nipples are frequently caused by incorrect attachment and/or thrush (see Section 3.3).

- Advise women of the indicators of good attachment, positioning and successful feeding:
  ○ audible and visible swallowing;
  ○ regular wet nappies;
  ○ breasts softening after a feed.

- Review a woman's experience with breastfeeding at each postnatal contact to identify any need for further support or intervention. This should form part of the documented and individualised postnatal care plan.

- All breastfeeding women should be shown how to hand express their colostrum or breast milk and be advised on safe storage.

- Advise women to avoid breast engorgement by frequent, unlimited feeding, simple analgesia, breast massage and hand expression if necessary. However, women should be advised to report promptly any signs and symptoms of mastitis, for example, flu-like symptoms or red, tender and painful breasts.

Further Resources

Baby Friendly Initiative. *Breastfeeding Research – an Overview*,
http://www.unicef.org.uk/BabyFriendly/News-and-Research/Research/Breastfeeding-research---An-overview/.

Baby Friendly Initiative. *Breastfeeding Care Pathway*,
http://www.unicef.org.uk/BabyFriendly/Health-Professionals/Care-Pathways/Breastfeeding/.

Postnatal Health Assessment

The Midwives Rules and Standards state that midwives should provide care to women and babies in the postnatal period for '*not less than 10 days and for such longer period as the midwife considers necessary*' (NMC 2012, p. 6). In recent years, the landscape of postnatal care has shifted significantly; for example, it is not uncommon for women to leave hospital within 6 hours following the birth of their baby (RCM 2014) or for community midwives to provide women with postnatal care within a clinic, rather than at the woman's home. In addition, the input of maternity support workers in the provision of routine postnatal care of mothers and babies has expanded greatly in some parts of the United Kingdom.

The healthcare professional responsible for performing the postnatal examination should aim to adopt a systematic and methodical approach that addresses *all* of the woman's and baby's needs, avoiding 'tick box' mentality based on physical markers alone. The central premise of the NICE (2006) quality standards for postnatal care is that a plan of individualised care is made with the woman, ideally during the antenatal period, which is clearly documented and reviewed frequently.

KEY POINTS

- Women want postnatal care that is responsive to their needs, is supportive and is based within their own homes (RCM 2014).

- Although women report overall satisfaction with their maternity care, postnatal care is the least satisfying experience, especially for primiparous women (Redshaw and Henderson 2015).

- All healthcare professionals involved in the care of mothers and babies should work within the relevant competencies developed by Skills for Health (NICE 2006).

ESSENTIALS OF MIDWIFERY CARE Current NICE guidelines (NICE 2006) (due for review in 2016) are comprehensive and a summary of the key advice that the healthcare professional should offer at each postnatal health assessment is provided below to aid revision:

- Ask the woman about her health and wellbeing, together with that of her baby. This should include making an assessment of common physical health problems and exploration of any symptoms reported by the woman or identified through clinical observations of mother and baby.

- Involve the woman in all aspects of her care. Offer consistent information and clear explanations that will facilitate the woman to monitor her health and that of her baby, and also recognise and report any concerns that relate to their physical, social or emotional health that may require investigation. This should include clear advice to the woman of the signs and symptoms of serious conditions, for example, postpartum haemorrhage (see Section 2.8), sepsis (see Section 4.5) and eclampsia (see Section 2.7).

- Enquire about women's emotional health and well-being, including a discussion of their support strategies and resolution of baby blues 10–14 days following birth (see Section 3.4).

- Advise women that topical cold therapy is effective at alleviating perineal discomfort and that paracetamol should be the first-line choice of analgesic.

- Organise the administration of anti-D immunoglobulin for a non-sensitised RhD-negative woman within 72 hours following the birth of an RhD-positive baby.

- Organise MMR vaccination for women before leaving the hospital/birth centre if previously identified during antenatal screening as being sero-negative for rubella.

- Be reassured that healthy babies:
  - Have normal colour for their ethnicity.
  - Maintain a stable body temperature.

- o Void urine and pass stools at regular intervals.
- o Are not tense, sleepy, floppy or excessively irritable and settle between feeds.
- Always refer babies who develop jaundice *less than 24 hours* following birth to a paediatrician. This is not a reassuring sign and may be indicative of sepsis, intestinal obstruction or fetomaternal blood group incompatibility (Blackburn 2013).
- Ensure that appropriate and timely newborn screening occurs in accordance with local and national guidelines:
  - o A complete, top-to-toe examination of the newborn occurs within 72 hours of birth by the appropriate healthcare professional.
  - o The newborn blood spot test that screens for a number of rare, but serious, conditions, including phenylketonuria, cystic fibrosis and maple syrup urine disease should be offered to parents when their baby is 5–8 days old. Since January 2015, this screening also includes rare inherited metabolic diseases (Public Health England 2012).
  - o A hearing screen should be completed before discharge from hospital/birth centre (or by week 4/5 in the community).
  - o Routine immunisations are organised as appropriate or recommended by the Department of Health, for example, BCG for babies born in areas with a high TB prevalence.
- Promote parent–baby attachment by:
  - o Advising parents and the wider family about their baby's social capabilities.
  - o Encouraging women to develop social networks that facilitate mother–baby interaction and support the transition to motherhood.
  - o Offering fathers information and support in adjusting to their new role and responsibilities within the new family unit.
- Inform parents that there is an association between co-sleeping and SIDS, especially where one or both parent smokes, consumes alcohol or uses drugs, and in low birth weight or pre-term babies.
- Advise parents that the use of cleansing agents/wipes, etc., on the newborn's skin/umbilical cord is not necessary.
- Advise parents that thrush should be treated with antifungal medication if the symptoms are causing pain to the woman or the baby or there are breastfeeding concerns. Note that persistent nappy rash is frequently caused by thrush.
- Evaluate the possible reasons for constipation and colic in a formula-fed baby, including feed preparation technique.

In addition, there are a number of specific elements of postnatal health assessment with which midwifery students need to become familiar. Some examples are offered in Table 1, alongside the relevant physiology that underpins the NICE (2006) recommendations, in order to aid clarity and encourage more detailed reading. This method could also serve as a useful revision tool.

PROFESSIONAL ACCOUNTABILITY A clear, individualised postnatal care plan for mother and baby should be clearly documented in order to facilitate continuity of midwifery care.

Further Resources

Skills for Health. *MCN4.*2015: *Assess the Health and Wellbeing of Women During the Postnatal Period,*
https://tools.skillsforhealth.org.uk/competence/show/html/id/3970/.

Table 1 Example of student revision tool for postnatal health assessment

NICE (2006) recommendation	Key physiology	Midwifery care
Daily assessment of uterine involution is not required	• Involution of the uterus involves three processes: contraction of the uterus, autolysis of myometrial cells and regeneration of the epithelium • The height of the fundus decreases by ˜1 cm per day and has normally descended into the true pelvis by around 10 days, when it can no longer be palpated abdominally • Involution is slower in multiparous women and is affected by mode of birth and infant feeding choice (Blackburn 2013)	• Involution of the uterus is unique to the individual woman and therefore daily palpation of the fundus is an unreliable tool to assess normal progress. In addition, intra-observer variability makes the measurement unreliable (Cluett *et al.* 1995) • Other factors can be more inductive of morbidity, e.g. pyrexia, offensive lochia and maternal well-being (Lewis 2007) • Providing women with information related to their postnatal health and well-being is likely to encourage self-reporting
The woman's first urine passed since birth should be documented	• Postnatal diuresis is the body's normal response to dissipating the increased extracellular fluid required during pregnancy • It usually occurs between days 2 and 5 postpartum, with fluid and electrolyte balance usually restored to pre-pregnant homeostasis by day 21 • Decreased bladder tone can be aggravated by instrumental delivery and prolonged labour. The pressure of the fetal head on the bladder may cause a transient loss of bladder sensation in the early postpartum days (Blackburn 2013)	• Atony (often as a result of a full bladder) is the most common cause of PPH (WHO 2012) • Reassure women that it is normal for them to void increased volumes of urine; this may be between 500 ml and 1 l • If women have not voided urine within 6 hours, efforts to assist include taking a warm bath or shower. Privacy is important and analgesia before voiding may be helpful. • Catheterisation should be considered beyond 6 hours. (NICE 2006; Blackburn 2013)
If jaundice develops in babies aged *24 hours and older*, its intensity should be monitored and systematically recorded	• Physiological jaundice is usually a normal process that occurs in the first few days following birth and is seen in 50–60% of term babies. It is a sign of bilirubin clearance. • Increased bilirubin production in the newborn is due to an increased circulating volume of red blood cells (and their subsequent destruction) • Visible jaundice usually appears when bilirubin levels reach 5–7 mg/dl • When bilirubin remains in the intestine, it is likely to be unconjugated. An early first feed and passage of meconium is therefore helpful in excreting bilirubin (Blackburn 2013)	• Monitor the baby's overall wellbeing with particular focus on hydration and alertness. • If a baby is significantly jaundiced on assessment or appears unwell, evaluation of the serum bilirubin level should be performed promptly and the postnatal care plan adjusted accordingly. • Always refer a baby who develops jaundice **less than 24 hours old** to a paediatrician. • Refer a baby to a paediatrician who first develops jaundice after 7 days; or who has prolonged jaundice beyond 14 days. (NICE 2006).

Mental Illness After Childbirth

It is usual for many women to experience an altered emotional state during the postnatal period and this is often linked to the physical and emotional demands of new motherhood. The challenge for the midwife is to be alert to the appearance of symptoms that may characterise a defined, serious mental health problem rather than an essentially normal response to motherhood. Given that 40% of women do not know the midwife who visits them postnatally and that one-third of women receive care from three or more midwives (Redshaw and Henderson 2015), this assessment can be a significant challenge.

KEY POINTS The Royal College of Psychiatrists offers comprehensive information to help support midwives in caring for women with altered postnatal mental health (RCP 2014). Some of this information is summarised below to aid revision:

- The *'baby blues'* is commonly experienced by over half of new mothers and is characterised by a range of emotions such as tearfulness, mood swings and anxiety. Symptoms usually appear by day 3 or 4 postpartum and should normally have disappeared by around day 10.
- *Postnatal depression* (PND) is a depressive illness that is characterised by a variety of symptoms indicative of low mood, including
    - depression;
    - irritability;
    - feelings of helplessness;
    - anxiety;
    - negative or guilty thoughts.
- Relatively common, the illness affects 10–15 women in 100 and the symptoms often appear at 1–2 months in the postpartum period.
- Women with PND may have thoughts of harming their babies, but it is rare for this to actually happen. However, it can be extremely distressing for women.
- Treatment depends on the severity of the depression and may be successfully managed by self-help interventions. Others may require anti-depressant medication and/or high-intensity psychological interventions such as CBT.
- Mindfulness-based cognitive therapy is associated with a significant reduction in both the incidence and reoccurrence of depression. It may also be an effective strategy for women who do not respond to other therapies, such as CBT (Segal *et al.* 2012).
- *Postpartum psychosis* is a psychiatric emergency that affects around 1 in 1000 women. It can start within days of giving birth and is characterised by a range of symptoms typically associated with other psychotic illness, including
    - rapid changes in mood;
    - behaving out of character;
    - losing inhibitions;
    - being 'manic';
    - severe confusion;
    - hallucinations and delusions.
- Women with a history of bipolar or schizoaffective disorders have a high risk of developing postpartum psychosis. The highest at-risk group is women who have experienced postpartum psychosis previously (50%) and women whose mothers or sisters have had postpartum psychosis (25%).
- Most women with postpartum psychosis require hospitalisation, ideally in a specialist mother and baby unit.

- Recovery can take 6–12 months and for most women, this is complete.
- In the 2014 MBRRACE report, 17% of the women who died had pre-existing mental health problems (Knight *et al.* 2014).

ESSENTIALS OF MIDWIFERY CARE
- NICE (2006) advises that:
  - At each postnatal visit, midwives should ask women about their emotional well-being, their family and social support and their usual coping strategies for dealing with day-to-day matters.
  - Women and their families/partners should be encouraged to discuss any changes in mood, emotional state and behaviour that are outside the woman's normal pattern with their midwife (or relevant healthcare professional, for example, health visitor).
  - At 10–14 days' postpartum, all women should be asked about resolution of 'baby blues' and further assessment/referral considered where indicated.
- The RCP (2014) suggests that the following advice can be helpful to offer women and their partners in alleviating the symptoms of postnatal depression:
  - joining groups/classes run for new parents;
  - making friends with other new parents;
  - not being afraid to tell their partners/friends about feeling depressed;
  - avoiding being 'superwoman';
  - maintaining a healthy diet and seeking exercise every day;
  - seeking help from voluntary organisations;
  - contacting their GP if the symptoms persist/worsen.
- NICE (2014) advises that:
  - Women who have pre-existing or new mental health illness need to be referred to a secondary mental health service, ideally a specialist perinatal mental health team, in order for a clear, written care plan to be made and disseminated as appropriate.
  - Women with mental health problems may have difficulties establishing a mother–baby relationship and therefore midwives need to be sensitive in supporting the establishment of that relationship.
- Ongoing clinical scrutiny of the woman is key to recognising deterioration.
- Midwives should ensure that they adhere to local and national guidelines for prompt referral of women at risk of developing postpartum psychosis or other mental health problem and communicate the urgency of that referral to the right professional.

PROFESSIONAL ACCOUNTABILITY
- Midwives should be aware of signs and symptoms of maternal mental health problems that may be experienced in the weeks and months following birth.
- Midwives have a clear responsibility under the NMC Code (NMC 2015) both to maintain the relevant skills required and to seek opportunities to develop them further.

Further Resources

Royal College of Psychiatrists. *Problems and Disorders*,
    http://www.rcpsych.ac.uk/healthadvice/problemsdisorders.aspx.

Association for Postnatal Illness,
http://apni.org/.

References

Ackerman, B. (2011) Infant feeding, in *Mayes' Midwifery*, 14th edn (eds S. Macdonald and J. Magill-Cuerden), Baillière Tindall Elsevier, Edinburgh, pp. 615–640.

BFI (2010) *Care Pathways: Breastfeeding, Baby Friendly Initiative*, http://www.unicef.org.uk/BabyFriendly/Health-Professionals/Care-Pathways/Breastfeeding/ (accessed 21 August 2015).

Blackburn, S.T. (2013) *Maternal, Fetal and Neonatal Physiology: a Clinical Perspective*, 4th edn, Elsevier Saunders, Maryland Heights, MO.

Borra, C., Iacovou, M. and Sevilla, A. (2015). New evidence on breastfeeding and postpartum depression: the importance of understanding women's intentions. *Maternal and Child Health Journal*, **19** (4), 897–907.

Cluett, E., Alexander, J. and Pickering, R. (1995) Is measuring postnatal symphysis–fundus distance worthwhile? *Midwifery*, **11** (4), 174–183.

Duijts, L., Jaddoe, V., Hofman, A. and Moll, A. (2010) Prolonged and exclusive breastfeeding reduces the risk of infectious diseases in infancy. *Pediatrics*, **126** (1), e18–e25.

Farrar, D., Tuffnell, D. and Ramage, C. (2014) Interventions for women in subsequent pregnancies following obstetric anal sphincter injury to reduce the risk of recurrent injury and associated harms. *Cochrane Database of Systematic Reviews*, Issue 11 (Art. No.: CD010374), doi: 10.1002/14651858.CD010374.pub2.

FSRH (2009) *Clinical Guidance: Postnatal Sexual and Reproductive Health, Faculty of Sexual and Reproductive* Healthcare, London.

Harder, T., Bergmann, R., Kallischnigg, G. and Plagemann, A. (2005) Duration of breastfeeding and risk of overweight: a meta-analysis. *American Journal of Epidemiology*, **162** (5), 397–403.

Knight, M., Kenyon, S., Brocklehurst, P., Neilson, J., Shakespeare, J. and Kurinczuk, J.J. (eds), on behalf of MBRRACE-UK (2014) *Saving Lives, Improving Mothers' Care – Lessons Learned to Inform Future Maternity Care from the UK and Ireland Confidential Enquiries into Maternal Deaths and Morbidity 2009–2012*, National Perinatal Epidemiology Unit, University of Oxford, Oxford.

Lawrence, R.A. and Lawrence, R.M. (1999) *Breastfeeding: a Guide for the Medical Profession*, Mosby, St Louis, MO.

Lewis, G. (ed.) (2007) The Confidential Enquiry into Maternal and Child Health *(CEMACH). Saving Mothers' Lives: Reviewing Maternal Deaths to Make Motherhood Safer – 2003–2005. The Seventh Report on Confidential Enquiries into Maternal Deaths in the United Kingdom*, CEMACH, London.

Liu, B., Jorm, L. and Banks, E. (2010) Parity, breastfeeding, and the subsequent risk of maternal type 2 diabetes. *Diabetes Care*, **33** (6), 1239–1241.

McAndrew, F., Thompson, J., Fellows, L., Large, A., Speed, M. and Renfrew, M. (2012) Infant Feeding Survey, *Health and Social Care Information* Centre, Leeds.

NICE (2006) *Postnatal Care*. National Institute for Health and Clinical Excellence, London.

NICE (2014) Antenatal and Postnatal Mental Health: Clinical Management and Service Guidance, *NICE Clinical Guideline CG192, National Institute for Health and Care* Excellence, London.

NMC (2012) *Midwives Rules and Standards*, Nursing and Midwifery Council, London.

NMC (2015) *The Code: Professional Standards of Practice and Behaviour for Nurses and Midwives*, Nursing and Midwifery Council, London.

Priddis, H., Schmied, V. and Dahlen, H. (2014) Women's experiences following severe perineal trauma: a qualitative study, *BMC Women's Health*, **14**, 32.

Public Health England (2012) Newborn Blood Spot Screening Programme: *Supporting Publications*, https://www.gov.uk/government/collections/newborn-blood-spot-screening-programme-supporting-publications (accessed 10 August 2015).

Rathfisch, G., Dikencik, B.K., Kizilkaya Beji, N., Comert, N., Tekirdag, A.I. and Kadioglu, A. (2010) Effects of perineal trauma on postpartum sexual function. *Journal of Advanced Nursing*, **66** (12), 2640–2649.

RCM (2014) Postnatal Care Planning: Pressure Points, Royal College of Midwives, London, https://www.rcm.org.uk/sites/default/files/Pressure%20Points%20-%20Postnatal%20Care%20Planning%20-%20Web%20Copy.pdf (accessed 10 August 2015).

RCP (2014) Postpartum Psychosis: Severe Mental Illness After Childbirth, Royal College of Psychiatrists, London, http://www.rcpsych.ac.uk/healthadvice/problemsdisorders/postpartumpsychosis.aspx (accessed 31 July 2015).

Redshaw, M. and Henderson, J. (2015) *Safely Delivered: a National Survey of Women's Experience of Maternity Care 2014*, National Perinatal Epidemiology Unit, University of Oxford, Oxford.

Segal, Z.V., Williams, J.M.G. and Teasdale, J.D. (2012) *Mindfulness-Based Cognitive Therapy for Depression*, 2nd edn, Guilford Press, New York.

UNICEF (2010) News: New Infant Feeding Survey Shows More Than 8 Out of 10 Babies Are Now Breastfed, http://www.unicef.org.uk/BabyFriendly/News-and-Research/News/New-infant-feeding-survey-says-more-than-8-out-of-10-babies-are-now-breastfed/ (accessed 10 August 2015).

WHO (2011) Statement: Exclusive Breastfeeding for Six Months Best for Babies Everywhere, http://www.who.int/mediacentre/news/statements/2011/breastfeeding&uscore;20110115/en/ (accessed 10 August 2015).

WHO (2012) WHO Recommendations for the Prevention and Treatment of Postpartum Haemorrhage, http://apps.who.int/iris/bitstream/10665/75411/1/9789241548502&uscore;eng.pdf (accessed 10 August 2015).

WHO/UNICEF (1989) *Ten steps to successful breastfeeding, in* Protecting, Supporting and Promoting Breastfeeding: the Special Role of Maternity Services, *a joint WHO/UNICEF statement*, World Health Organization, Geneva.

World Cancer Research Fund/American Institute for Cancer Research (2010) Continuous Update Project: Keeping the Science Current – Breast Cancer 2010 Report: Food, Nutrition, Physical Activity, and the Prevention of Breast Cancer, http://www.wcrf.org/sites/default/files/Breast-Cancer-2010-Report.pdf (accessed 10 August 2015).

PART IV

Hot Topics

Breech Birth

The number of breech presentation babies born vaginally has dwindled significantly in recent years and particularly coincided with the increasing use of ultrasound, electronic fetal heart rate monitoring and a rapid rise in caesarean section rates. Consequently, the skill set of midwives and obstetricians in supporting vaginal breech birth has been eroded over time. The term breech trial (Hannah *et al.* 2000) concluded that caesarean section was the safest mode of delivery for breech babies and, consequently, attitudes and practice changed almost immediately. A number of studies have subsequently demonstrated that the outcomes of vaginal breech deliveries are comparable to those of planned caesarean sections, the largest of these being the PREMODA group study (Goffinet *at al.* 2006). The key factors in this study were familiarity with routine, vaginal breech birth together with strict risk assessment.

The current RCOG guidelines (RCOG 2006) advise that the safest mode of delivery for term babies presenting by the breech is planned caesarean section; however, this guideline is currently being reviewed and the revised version is due to be published in 2016. New guidance is timely given the increasing debate and growing evidence from a number of midwives and obstetricians around the United Kingdom who report good outcomes from vaginal breech birth.

It is important to distinguish between a spontaneous vaginal breech birth and vaginal breech delivery. As midwives are most likely to encounter women who choose the former (or who present with an undiagnosed breech), this will chiefly be described below.

KEY POINTS

- Breech presentation occurs in 3–4% of all pregnancies (RCOG 2006), although up to one-third are not diagnosed before labour.
- NICE (2012) recommends that women with an uncomplicated breech presentation should be offered external cephalic version from 36 weeks' gestation.
- Breech presentation has a number of variants:
    - *Extended* or frank, where the thighs are flexed and the legs extended at the knees and alongside the trunk. This is the most common breech presentation in primigravidae and results in a well-fitting presenting part.
    - *Flexed* or complete, where the fetus sits ('tailor' sitting) with thighs and knees flexed and feet close to the buttocks. This is more common in multigravidae and the presenting part will be poorly applied. Key risks are cord prolapse **(see Section 2.6)** and early rupture of the membranes.
    - *Footling*, where one or both feet are below the buttocks and hips and the knees are extended. This is comparatively rare and more common with pre-term babies, and it also results in an ill-fitting presenting part.
    - *Knee presentation*, where one or both knees are below the buttocks, with one or both hips extended and the knees flexed. This is the least common breech presentation (Lewis 2011b).
- Breech birth is more likely to occur where:
    - Onset of labour is spontaneous.
    - Normal progress during the first stage of labour occurs.
    - Augmentation is not used.
    - Non-pharmacological analgesia is used.
    - A birth environment conducive to promoting normality is maintained (see Section 2.1.2).
    - Normal progress and descent occur during the second stage and spontaneous pushing is encouraged (Evans 2012a).

ESSENTIAL PHYSIOLOGY

- The optimal position for the fetus to enter the pelvis is right sacroanterior (RSA).
- When the fetus meets the resistance of the pelvic floor, it will rotate to right sacrolateral (RSL).
- With further descent, the anterior buttock will be visible.
- The baby's hips flex laterally as the buttocks pivot under the symphysis pubis and rumping occurs (the widest diameter of the buttocks is born).
- Restitution occurs.
- The baby will rotate to RSA then direct sacroanterior (SA) as the shoulders enter the pelvis.
- With further descent and arching of the baby's back as it moves under the symphysis pubis, the legs are born.
- As the baby descends and continues to rotate into position, the effect of uterine contractions on the spine initiates the Perez reflex:
  - The head and back arch backwards, which moves the head out from underneath the symphysis pubis.
  - The baby will pass urine, which also empties the bladder of amniotic fluid and decreases the abdominal volume and thus circumference, facilitating passage through the birth canal.
- The baby will now rotate to LSA and this enables the head to enter the pelvis and releases the anterior shoulder.
- It will then return to direct SA, releasing the posterior shoulder and aligning the head for birth.
- In order to flex its head onto its chest, the baby will perform a tummy tuck, which will compel the mother to move forwards, bringing her pelvis over the baby's face as it is born. (Lewis 2011b; Evans 2012a,b).

ESSENTIALS OF MIDWIFERY CARE Evans (2012a,b) offers comprehensive advice for supporting vaginal breech birth, a summary of which is offered below to aid revision:

- An upright kneeling position enhances rotation and descent and many women will spontaneously adopt this position during labour. This means that the baby should have its back to the mother's front (or 'tum to bum'). Although not ideal, if the woman is in the supine position, the same key principles apply:
  - don't panic;
  - hands off the breech;
  - look for rotation and descent;
  - aim to keep baby back to front.
- Do not interfere with the spontaneous movements that the woman makes as these facilitate a physiological birth. For example, she may spontaneously sit back on her heels to widen the pelvis and encourage descent and flexion of the head.
- Monitor the woman's progress carefully throughout. If contractions cease, this should be respected as it usually indicates a problem that requires intervention.
- Monitor the fetal heart as for any other birth.
- Adopt a hands-off approach (including leaving any faecal matter *in situ*) until the shoulders have been born and then gently support the baby's weight as the head emerges.

- Be reassured where:
  - The baby's colour is bluish, not white or mottled.
  - The baby has good tone, for example pointy toes and clenched hands.
  - The cord is plump and perfused.
  - There is a cord 'valley' or chest cleavage – this indicates that the arms are flexed.
- Be alert when the:
  - Cord valley is absent or the chest is barrel-shaped – this indicates that the arms are extended.
  - Perineum appears 'full' after the arms have been born – this indicates a flexed head.
  - Baby's chest is bulging towards you – this may indicate an extended head.

Usually there is no need to intervene with a spontaneous breech birth. However, if the baby's arms are up alongside its head or the head does not flex, there are some simple manoeuvres to help, the simplest being to press on the maternal iliac crests to alter the shape of the pelvis.

- *Nuchal arms*:
  - Generally only occur when the fetus enters the pelvis LSA.
  - Adopt 'prayer hands' – place fingers on the baby's ribs and shoulder blades and apply even pressure.
  - Slight lift to disimpact.
  - Rotate the baby 180°, taking its front around the maternal back if possible. This will release the anterior arm.
  - Rotate the baby 90° back the other way into the SA position. This will release the other arm.
  - Alternatively, the baby can be rotated 270°, taking the sacrum posteriorly.
- *Deflexed head*:
  - Using a middle finger, push the occiput to bring the head forwards.
  - Alternatively, hold the baby gently round the shoulders and pivot its body back, away from the sacrum. Maintain the hold, allowing the head to stretch the perineal tissue (Frank's nudge[1]).
  - A *persistent deflexed head* will require the modified Mauriceau–Smellie–Veit manoeuvre:
    - Wait until the nape of the neck is visible.
    - Place a middle finger on the occiput, and the first and third fingers of the other hand on the baby's cheekbones.
    - When hands are in place, ask the mother to drop forwards and assist the birth of the head, following the curve of Carus.
- *Extended head*:
  - Holding the baby gently round the shoulders, press both thumbs into the sub-clavicular space and lift slightly to bring the shoulders forwards.
  - Repeat two or three times if necessary to bring the head down.
  - Hold the baby slightly back from the sacrum to maintain flexion and allow the perineal tissue to stretch (Frank's nudge).
  - An assistant can apply suprapubic pressure.

---

[1] After Professor Frank Louwen, University Hospital Frankfurt.

PROFESSIONAL ACCOUNTABILITY

- Midwives must respond calmly and appropriately to an unexpected breech birth. Courage and communication are essential components of care.
- As with all aspects of midwifery, good documentation is an essential requirement of safe and effective practice.
- An awareness of the impact of undiagnosed breech birth on women and their partners needs to be clearly recognised and appropriate action taken, including debriefing.

Further Resources

Cardinal movements of the breech baby, https://www.youtube.com/watch?v=l16dPHaOGj0.

Domestic Abuse

Women's Aid defines domestic violence as 'physical, psychological, sexual or financial violence that takes place within an intimate or family-type relationship and forms a pattern of coercive and controlling behaviour'. The term 'domestic abuse' is also used in the literature as domestic violence often includes other types of abusive behaviours that may not involve actual physical harm, such as bullying, withholding money and telephone calls or destructive criticism. The human and economic cost of domestic abuse is so great that even marginally effective interventions can be cost-effective and therefore justified (NICE 2014).

KEY POINTS

- Domestic abuse is common and affects one in four women in their lifetime, regardless of ethnicity, social class or lifestyle. However, vulnerability to abuse is associated with social exclusion (Walby and Allen 2004).

- Pregnancy is a known trigger for the onset of domestic abuse. In the 2011 'Saving Mothers' Lives' report (Lewis 2011a), 11 women were murdered, most of whom were pregnant.

- Domestic violence increases the risk of miscarriage, pre-term labour and maternal and fetal injuries (Baird and Mitchell 2013).

- Two women per week are killed by their partners or former partners (ONS 2015).

- All forms of domestic abuse stem from the abuser's desire for power and control over an intimate partner or other family member.

- Domestic abuse is most commonly experienced by women and perpetrated by men.

- Men can also experience violence from their partners, both gay and straight. However, women's violence towards men is frequently self defence and is rarely defined by consistent patterns of controlling and coercive behaviour (Women's Aid 2015).

- Indicators of domestic abuse include:
  - Anxiety and depression; sleep disorders.
  - Substance abuse.
  - Pelvic pain, sexual dysfunction, repeated urinary tract infections.
  - Adverse pregnancy outcomes, for example, miscarriage, terminations, pre-term labour and stillbirth.
  - Vaginal bleeding.
  - Sexually acquired infections (Black 2011).

ESSENTIALS OF MIDWIFERY CARE NICE (2014) has developed a number of key recommendations that are based on the premise that working collaboratively with relevant multi-agency professionals is key to tackling the issue at both operational and strategic levels. A summary of these recommendations is offered below:

- Creating an environment that facilitates safe disclosure of abuse, for example, by displaying accessible information in antenatal clinic waiting rooms that clearly signposts sources of help and support.

- Ensuring that trained, frontline staff ask women about domestic abuse:
  - It is good practice to ask all women routinely during pregnancy if they have experienced abuse, even if no indicators of abuse exist.
  - Opportunities for women to be seen on their own and in privacy should therefore be facilitated.

- Providing specific training for health and social care staff in how to respond effectively to domestic abuse, thereby providing a universal response. For midwives, this means:
  - an understanding of the dynamics of domestic abuse;
  - responding to a woman with compassion and understanding;
  - assessment of a woman's immediate safety and referral to specialist services;
  - ensuring that the processes for sharing information do not put the woman at further risk.
- At the end of the postnatal period, the coordinating healthcare professional should ensure that the woman's physical, emotional and social well-being is reviewed. This should include an opportunity to screen for domestic abuse (NICE 2006).

ADDITIONAL EVIDENCE POINTS NICE (2014):

- There is currently insufficient evidence to make recommendations about programmes that prevent domestic abuse.
- Working in a multi-agency partnership is the most effective way to approach the issue at operational and strategic levels.
- Initial and ongoing training with support is required for all staff.

PROFESSIONAL ACCOUNTABILITY

- It may be necessary for midwives to share information with other agencies when a woman discloses abuse, and this can be complex if there are children involved.
- The principles of consent, confidentiality and data protection must be upheld.
- The Calidicott Guardian principles can support midwives in this important aspect of their practice.

Further Resources

Women's Aid, http://www.womensaid.org.uk.

Refuge, http://www.refuge.org.uk/who-we-are/.

Obesity

Obesity is an increasing problem within society that has far-reaching and serious consequences for many aspects of health, including women's reproductive health. The 2013
Health Survey for England (HSCIC 2014) identified that 33% of women were overweight
and 24% obese. NICE (2010) defines a woman who is overweight as one who has a body
mass index (BMI) of 25–29.9 kg/m^2. An obese woman is defined as having a BMI greater
than or equal to 30 kg/m^2.

KEY POINTS

- NICE calculates obesity health risk from BMI and waist measurement. When this calculation is applied to the Health Survey data, more than half of the women were in the
  increased, high- or very high-risk categories.
- Maternal obesity has a known association with thrombosis and thromboembolism, the
  leading cause of direct maternal deaths (Knight *et al.* 2014).
- Over 22% of the women who died as recorded in the most recent MBRRACE report
  (Knight *et al.* 2014) were overweight and 27% were obese, consistent with the data
  reported from the Health Survey for England.
- Obesity is independently associated with higher odds of dying from specific pregnancy
  complications (Nair *et al.* 2015).
- Overweight and obese women are more at risk of caesarean section (Dignon and Truslove
  2013), gestational diabetes and macrosomia (Sebire *et al.* 2001), together with associated sequelae such as shoulder dystocia. They are also less likely to initiate and sustain
  breastfeeding (Amir and Donath 2007).

ESSENTIALS OF MIDWIFERY CARE

- Maternal obesity is a public health problem, not an isolated maternity issue, and therefore
  partnership working with community public health services is essential when developing
  interventions for maternal obesity (Heslehurst *et al.* 2011).
- Do not advise women to begin a weight-loss programme during pregnancy because of
  the risks to fetal health and well-being (NICE 2010).
- Joint CMACE/RCOG (2010) guidelines include detailed recommendations for the care of
  overweight and obese women during childbirth. These are based on the principles of
  effective, collaborative care and risk assessment. Some examples include:
  - Women with a BMI of 30 and above should be assessed throughout pregnancy for the
    risk of thromboembolism and appropriate prophylaxis regimes applied to their care.
  - An appropriately sized cuff should be used for BP measurement and the correct size
    documented in the woman's notes.
  - Wherever possible, normal birth should be encouraged and continuous midwifery care
    during labour facilitated. Obesity alone is not an indication for induction of labour.
  - For women with a BMI of 40 and above, midwives need to liaise closely with all mem-
    bers of the multi-professional team, including anaesthetists and operating department
    staff.
- NICE (2010) has developed a number of recommendations for midwifery practice. These
  include:
  - Ensuring that midwives have the necessary communication techniques to discuss
    weight management and risks in a sensitive manner.
  - Advising pregnant women that a healthy diet and being physically active are of benefit
    to themselves and their unborn babies and will also facilitate the achievement of a
    healthy weight after giving birth.

- Giving practical advice about keeping physically active during pregnancy, for example, swimming and brisk walking are both safe and beneficial.
- Offering women with a BMI of 30 or more referral to a dietician at booking.

ADDITIONAL EVIDENCE POINTS CMACE/RCOG (2010):

- Maternal obesity is one of the most common risk factors in maternity care.
- Obesity is associated with a range of serious adverse outcomes.

PROFESSIONAL ACCOUNTABILITY In line with the NMC Code (NMC 2015), midwives must work to coordinate safe and effective maternity care of overweight and obese women within the multi-professional team. This includes working within locally and nationally agreed integrated care pathways.

Further Resources

Public Health England. *Maternal Obesity*,
    https://www.noo.org.uk/NOO_about_obesity/maternal_obesity.

Royal College of Midwives. *Obesity*,
    https://www.rcm.org.uk/tags/obesity.

Recognising the Deteriorating Woman

MBRRACE, in their recent 'Saving Lives, Improving Mothers' Care' report (Knight *et al.* 2014), state that the early identification of pregnant and postnatal women whose medical condition is deteriorating, along with rapid actions to diagnose and treat them, *will save lives*. This highlights the importance of routine measurements such as pulse, temperature, respiratory rate and blood pressure.

Midwives are at the forefront of maternity care and as such a deteriorating woman will usually present first to a midwife. The midwife has a critical part to play in recognising the deteriorating woman and acting upon this in a suitable and timely manner.

KEY POINTS

- There were 321 maternal deaths from direct (an obstetric complication) or indirect (a previous existing disease) causes in 2009–2012 in the United Kingdom (Knight *et al.* 2014).

- In 52% of the cases of maternal death included in the MBRRACE report (Knight *et al.* 2014), it was identified that improvements to care might have made a difference to the outcome.

- Reasons for substandard care included:
  - failure to recognise the deteriorating woman;
  - ineffective diagnosis of the condition;
  - Ineffective or incorrect treatment;
  - poor communication within the multi-disciplinary team (Knight *et al.* 2014).

- In several cases, inadequate observations were made or abnormal observations were not escalated appropriately.

- Almost one-quarter of women who died had sepsis. Knight *et al.* (2014) highlight that prompt diagnosis and treatment of sepsis can make the difference between life and death (see Section 4.5).

ESSENTIALS OF MIDWIFERY CARE

- Although midwives may not be familiar with some of the complex conditions with which women present, the basics of effective care require skills and ability in simple measures, such as the ABCDE approach (Raynor 2012). Taking a history and undertaking assessment of vital signs are the starting point, regardless of the presenting health issue (Raynor 2012).

- The MBRRACE report (Knight *et al.* 2014) states: 'All women with any symptoms or signs of ill health, including those who are postnatal, should have a full set of basic observations taken (temperature, pulse rate, respiratory rate and blood pressure) and the results documented and acted upon. Normality cannot be presumed without measurement'.

- Churchill *et al.* (2014) drive home the importance of 'Think Sepsis', a key take-home message from their report. They state that the key actions for diagnosis and management of sepsis are:
  - timely recognition;
  - rapid administration of intravenous antibiotics;
  - quick involvement of experts, with senior review being essential.

- Although a key observation, respiration rate is inconsistently recorded in maternity care (Raynor 2012). However, the respiration rate is an early indicator of acute critical illness, including sepsis (McBride *et al.* 2005; Raynor 2012). Subtle changes in this vital sign will be seen much earlier than others, such as blood pressure (Lewis 2007). Therefore, it is essential that respiration rate is recorded as part of routine care, in order to establish a baseline for each woman and thereby enabling recognition of a deviation from normal ranges.

- A midwife should be alert to any changes in a woman's condition and escalate such changes in a timely manner.
- Use of a MEOWS (Modified Early Obstetric Warning Score) chart aims to enable early recognition of the deteriorating woman and is currently recommended by the RCOG (2011) based on NICE (2007) guidance. However, the evidence base behind its use is lacking and the recommendation is based on informal consensus rather than evidence (RCOG 2011).
- Martin and Hutchon (2008) highlighted the need for a national MEOWS chart.

PROFESSIONAL ACCOUNTABILITY

- Midwives must be competent in recording vital signs and observing maternal well-being.
- In addition, the importance of interdisciplinary team work and communication cannot be underestimated.
- MEOWS charts should be used appropriately, completed fully and trigger scores totalled in every case. Results should be escalated as required according to the scoring system.

Further Resources

Knight, M., Kenyon, S., Brocklehurst, P., Neilson, J., Shakespeare, J. and Kurinczuk, J.J. (eds), on behalf of MBRRACE-UK (2014) *Saving Lives, Improving Mothers' Care – Lessons Learned to Inform Future Maternity Care from the UK and Ireland Confidential Enquiries into Maternal Deaths and Morbidity 2009–2012*, National Perinatal Epidemiology Unit, University of Oxford, Oxford.

Sepsis

Infection is a serious and potentially life-threatening complication of the perinatal period that should never be underestimated. Healthy women can deteriorate rapidly and, even where there is prompt recognition and treatment, morbidly and mortality risks are high. In the latest MBRACCE report (Knight *et al*. 2014), maternal sepsis is identified as the leading cause of maternal death, with absent or incomplete maternal observations a particular feature of postnatal care. This includes women who died from genital tract sepsis, influenza and pneumococcal disease. Women are equally at risk during pregnancy and therefore this section is not confined to the puerperium alone.

KEY POINTS Churchill *et al*. (2014) offer comprehensive information and detail in their report:

- Pregnant women are uniquely at risk from sepsis owing to modulation of their immune system. Sepsis and its accompanying systemic inflammatory response syndrome (SIRS) reflect the inability of the body to regulate the immune system.

- Septic shock occurs in cases of severe infection caused by bacterial toxins that are released into the circulation. These toxins trigger a massive inflammatory immune response and, because this response is poorly controlled, multiple organ damage will ultimately occur.

- Pregnant and postpartum women may appear well until the point of collapse, as the pregnancy-induced challenges to their immune system enable them to withstand physiological insult for longer than usual.

- Alterations in baseline observations of temperature, pulse, respirations and blood pressure are frequently seen in early sepsis development and should therefore not be ignored.

- Risk factors for maternal sepsis include:
  - obesity;
  - diabetes;
  - anaemia;
  - history of pelvic infection;
  - history of group B infection;
  - amniocentesis;
  - cervical cerclage or other invasive procedures;
  - prolonged spontaneous rupture of membranes and close contact with group A streptococcal (GAS) infection.

- In the most recent MBRACCE report (Knight *et al*. 2014), maternal deaths from genital tract sepsis have declined significantly. However, other infections remain significant, in particular *influenza*:
  - Influenza is highly infectious and is transmitted via nasopharyngeal secretions with a usual incubation period of 1–3 days.
  - There are three types of influenza virus, with influenza A and B being responsible for most clinical illness.
  - Symptoms include fever, headache, anorexia, myalgia, profound malaise and minor respiratory symptoms.
  - 36 maternal deaths from influenza were reported, most due to the subtype A virus H1N1, commonly known as swine flu.

- The principles of effective treatment for sepsis are:
  - timely recognition;
  - prompt administration of antibiotics;
  - involvement of senior clinicians (Churchill *et al*. 2014).

- Poor communication between the healthcare team has been identified as a contributory factor in some maternal deaths. This included junior medical staff not informing their more senior colleagues and midwives failing to recognise signs of a deteriorating woman.

ESSENTIALS OF MIDWIFERY CARE Churchill *et al.* (2014) outline the key messages for midwives and health providers in the MBRRACE report. Their recommendations and those provided by the RCOG (2012) Green-top Guideline include the following:

- Discuss the benefits of influenza vaccination with pregnant women and promote its uptake at all stages during pregnancy (Public Health England 2013).
- The midwife should make all women aware of the severity of influenza in pregnancy.
- Antiviral treatment should be commenced as early as possible in pregnant women with signs of influenza, ideally within the first 48 hours of the onset of symptoms.
- Midwives need to raise awareness of the signs and symptoms of sepsis and urge women to seek medical assessment.
- Women presenting with signs of sepsis should be referred for medical review as a matter of urgency.
- The symptoms of sepsis may be non-specific and women may present with vague symptoms. Midwives should have a high index of suspicion if women report malaise, non-specific pain, loose stools or diarrhoea and occasional vomiting.
- A thorough clinical history should be taken, including signs of otitis media or sinusitis. Pelvic and rectal pain or discharge should also be investigated.
- Clinical signs suggestive of sepsis include one or more of the following:
  - pyrexia;
  - hypothermia;
  - tachycardia;
  - tachypnoea;
  - hypoxia;
  - hypotension;
  - oliguria;
  - impaired consciousness and failure to respond to treatment;
  - upper respiratory tract symptoms and sore throat should also alert the midwife.
- Always '*think sepsis*' (Churchill *et al.* 2014, p. 27) when a pregnant or recently pregnant woman presents as unwell. Be alert to women who present repeatedly to antenatal or postnatal clinics.
- Take a full set of observations (temperature, pulse, blood pressure and respirations) from any woman who presents with symptoms of ill health. All vital signs should be recorded on a Modified Early Obstetric Warning Score (MEOWS) chart. Document the findings and act on them (NICE 2006).
- Base care on the 'sepsis six' care bundle (UK Sepsis Trust 2013):
  - Obtain an arterial blood gas and administer high flow oxygen.
  - Obtain blood cultures.
  - Commence IV antibiotics.
  - Commence IV fluid resuscitation.
  - Obtain blood for Hb and lactate.
  - Monitor hourly urine output.

PROFESSIONAL ACCOUNTABILITY It is recommended that education on the recognition and treatment of sepsis be incorporated into mandatory training, particularly in low-risk maternity settings (Churchill *et al.* 2014).

Further Resources

UK Sepsis Trust. *Samantha's Story*, http://sepsistrust.org/story/samantha/ (accessed 1 December 2015).

References

Amir, L.H. and Donath, S. (2007) A systematic review of maternal obesity and breastfeeding intention, initiation and duration. *BMC Pregnancy and Childbirth*, **7**, 9.

Baird, K. and Mitchell, T. (2013) Issues for consideration by researchers conducting sensitive research with women who have endured domestic violence during pregnancy. *Evidence Based Midwifery*, **11** (1), 21–27.

Black, M.C. (2011). Intimate partner violence and adverse health consequences: implications for clinicians. *American Journal of Lifestyle Medicine*, **5** (5), 428–439.

Churchill, D., Rodger, A., Clift, J. and Tuffnell, D. (2014) *Think sepsis, in Saving Lives, Improving Mothers' Care – Lessons Learned to Inform Future Maternity Care from the UK and Ireland Confidential Enquiries into Maternal Deaths and Morbidity* 2009–2012 (eds M. Knight, S. Kenyon, P. Brocklehurst, N. Neilson, J. Shakespeare and J.J. Kurinczuk, on behalf of MBRRACE-UK), National Perinatal Epidemiology Unit, University of Oxford, Oxford, pp. 27–43.

CMACE/RCOG (2010) *Joint Guideline: Management of Women with Obesity in Pregnancy*, https://www.rcog.org.uk/globalassets/documents/guidelines/cmacercogjointguidelinemana-gementwomenobesitypregnancya.pdf (accessed June 2015).

Dignon, A. and Truslove, T. (2013) Obesity, pregnancy outcomes and caesarean section: a structured review of the combined literature. *Evidence Based Midwifery*, **11** (4), 132–137.

Evans, J. (2012a) Understanding physiological breech birth. *Essentially MIDIRS*, **3** (2), 17–21.

Evans, J. (2012b) The final piece of the breech birth jigsaw? *Essentially MIDIRS*, **3** (3): 46–49.

Goffinet, F., Caravol, M., Foidart, J., Alexander,S., Uzan, S., Subtil, D. and Bréart, G., and PREMODA Study Group (2006) Is planned vaginal delivery for breech presentation at term still an option? Results of an observational prospective survey in France and Belgium. *American Journal of Obstetrics and Gynaecology*, **194** (4), 1002–1011.

Hannah, M., Hannah, W., Hewson, S., Hodnett, E., Saigal, S. and Willan, A. (2000) Planned caesarean section versus planned vaginal birth for breech presentation at term: a randomised multicentre trial. *The Lancet*, **356** (9239), 1375–1383.

Heslehurst, N., Moore, H., Rankin, J., Ells, L.J., Wilkinson, J.R. and Summberbell, C.D. (2011) How can maternity services be developed to effectively address maternal obesity? A qualitative study. *Midwifery*, **27** (5), 170–177.

HSCIC (2014) *Health Survey for England 2013, Health and Social Care Information* Centre, Leeds.

Knight, M., Kenyon, S., Brocklehurst, P., Neilson, J., Shakespeare, J. and Kurinczuk, J.J. (eds), on behalf of MBRRACE-UK (2014) *Saving Lives, Improving Mothers' Care – Lessons Learned to Inform Future Maternity Care from the UK and Ireland Confidential Enquiries into Maternal Deaths and Morbidity 2009–2012*, National Perinatal Epidemiology Unit, University of Oxford, Oxford.

Lewis,G. (ed.) (2007) *The Confidential Enquiry into Maternal and Child Health (CEMACH). Saving Mothers' Lives: Reviewing Maternal Deaths to Make Motherhood Safer – 2003–2005. The Seventh Report on Confidential Enquiries into Maternal Deaths in the United Kingdom*, CEMACH, London.

Lewis, G. (ed.) (2011a) Saving Mothers' Lives: Reviewing Maternal Deaths to Make Motherhood Safer: 2006–2008 The Eighth Report of the Confidential Enquiries into Maternal Deaths in the United Kingdom. *Centre for Maternal and Child Enquiries (CMACE), London; BJOG, 2011*, **118** (Suppl 1), 1–203.

Lewis, P. (2011b) Malpositions and malpresentations, in *Mayes' Midwifery*, 14th edn (eds S. Macdonald and J. Magill-Cuerden), Baillière Tindall Elsevier, Edinburgh, pp. 869–897.

Martin, W. and Hutchon, S. (2008) Multidisciplinary training in obstetric critical care. *Best Practice and Research. Clinical Obstetrics and Gynaecology*, **22** (5), 953–964.

McBride, J., Knight, D., Piper, J. and Smith, G.B. (2005) Long-term effect of introducing an early warning score on respiratory rate charting on general wards. *Resuscitation*, **65**, 41–44.

Nair, M., Kurinczuk, J.J., Brocklehurst, P., Sellers, S., Lewis, G. and Knight, M. (2015) Factors associated with maternal death from direct pregnancy complications: a UK national case–control study. *British Journal of Obstetrics and Gynaecology*, **122** (5), 653–622.

NICE (2006) *Postnatal Care*. National Institute for Health and Clinical Excellence, London.

NICE (2007) Acutely Ill Patients in Hospital: Recognition of and Response to Acute Illness in Adults in Hospital, *NICE Clinical Guideline CG50, National Institute for Health and Clinical* Excellence, London.

NICE (2010) *Weight Management Before, During and After Pregnancy*, NICE Public Health Guidance PH27, National Institute for Health and Clinical Excellence, London.

NICE (2012) *Quality Statement 11: Fetal Wellbeing – External Cephalic Version*, NICE Quality Standard QS22, National Institute for Health and Clinical Excellence, London.

NICE (2014) *Domestic Violence and Abuse: How Health Services, Social Care and the Organisations They Work With Can Respond Effectively*, NICE Public Health Guidance PH50, National Institute for Health and Care Excellence, London.

NMC (2015) *The Code: Professional Standards of Practice and Behaviour for Nurses and Midwives*, Nursing and Midwifery Council, London.

ONS (2015) *Crime Statistics, Focus on Violent Crime and Sexual Offences, 2013/14, Office for National Statistics*, http://www.ons.gov.uk/ons/rel/crime-stats/crime-statistics/focus-on-violent-crime-and-sexual-offences--2013-14/index.html (accessed 21 August 2015).

Public Health England (2013) *Immunisation Against Infectious Disease. The Green Book*, https://www.gov.uk/government/uploads/system/uploads/attachment_data/file/266583/The_Green_book_front_cover_and_contents_page_December_2013.pdf, (accessed 10 August 2015].

Raynor, M.D. (2012) Recognition of the critically ill woman, in *Midwifery Practice: Critical Illness, Complications and Emergencies Case Book* (eds M.D. Raynnor, J.E. Marshall and K. Jackson), Open University Press, Maidenhead, pp. 5–18.

RCOG (2006) *The Management of Breech Presentation*, Green-top Guideline No. 20b, Royal College of Obstetricians and Gynaecologists, London.

RCOG (2011) *Maternal Collapse in Pregnancy and the Puerperium*, Green-top Guideline No. 56, Royal College of Obstetricians and Gynaecologists, London.

RCOG (2012) Bacterial Sepsis in Pregnancy, *Green-top Guideline No 64a*, Royal College of Obstetricians andGynaecologists, London.

Sebire, N., Jolly, M., Harris, J., Wadsworth, J., Joffe, M., Beard, R.W., Regan, L. and Robinson, S. (2001). Maternal obesity and pregnancy outcome: a study of 287,213 pregnancies in London. *International Journal of Obesity and Related Metabolic Disorders: Journal of the International Association for the Study of Obesity*, **25** (8), 1175–1182.

UK Sepsis Trust (2013) *Clinical Toolkits*, http://sepsistrust.org/clinical-toolkit/ (accessed 1 December 2015).

Walby, S. and Allen, J. (2004) *Domestic Violence, Sexual Assault and Stalking: Findings from the British Crime Survey*, Home Office Research, Development and Statistics Directorate, London.

Women's Aid (2015) https://www.womensaid.org.uk/information-support/what-is-domestic-abuse-2/ (accessed 1 December 2015).

Conclusion: Top Tips for Examination Success

Dr Martin Spurin

Exams? Do you hate them? Even the word can send a shudder down the spine. If you feel like this, don't worry as you're not alone. There are a few reasons why students do not do well in exams, and I will address two of them here. The first is about how students prepare for the exam; the second is how they are in the actual exam.

Preparation - Revision

You need to start by believing that you deserve to do well in the exam, otherwise you will not commit yourself to it. The preparation can start weeks in advance. You start by reading all your notes and then, as the exam approaches, intensify your revision and then devote more time to your notes. It is always best to try and get hold of past exam papers in your module so that you can get a feel for its style.

But you might have done all this before and still not have done very well. At this stage, it is therefore worth trying something different. A lot of exams are about testing your short-term memory; therefore, it may be strategic to enhance recall that you need to improve. To help us understand this and other aspects of exam preparation, let us apply the work of O'Connor and Seymour (1990).

When we process information in our minds, we rely on a strategy. A strategy is essentially how you organise your thoughts and behaviour to accomplish a task. When it comes to revision, therefore, you might just be using the wrong strategy. To illustrate, read the following quickly and as you do, count how many 'f's are in the following sentence:

Finished files are the result of years of scientific study combined

with the experience of many years

There are, of course, six 'f's in the sentence. If you got that right then well done; you probably used the right strategy (unless of course you've seen it before and just remembered it). If you got less than six, then you may have used the wrong strategy. There is a belief that three of the strategies we use are visual, auditory and kinaesthetic. If you only counted three 'f's in the sentence, it is likely that you used an auditory system; in other words, you listened for the 'f's. The problem with this is that words such as 'of' tend to get passed over and the 'f' in the word does not really sound like an 'f'. An auditory strategy doe not really work, so it is important to try another one. The same applies to memorising information. The interesting thing is that our eyes often indicate which system we are using:

- *Visual*. Here we think in pictures or stories. When we use visual memory, unless we are left handed, we tend to look up to the left. Try thinking of the colour of your neighbour's garage.
- *Auditory*. We use this when we are listening and trying to memorise words. When we do this, we tend to look sideways. Imagine listening to a strange sound late at night.
- *Kinaesthetic*. Here we try to feel what we are thinking. Think about the thoughts you had when you were last upset; chances are you looked down with your eyes.

We do tend to favour and use one of these strategies more than the others. We also tend to get on better and communicate more effectively with others who also share the same strategy. If you find that you prefer one lecturer's style of teaching, it might be that they are a visual type of person like you and so are always painting mental pictures to explain themselves. You relate well to this, and that is why you understand them better.

Trying a Different Strategy

Let us take spelling as an example. One reason why people are poor at spelling is that they often rely on an auditory system. They listen to the sound of the word in their mind and then spell it. Yet a large percentage of English words do not spell like they sound. You cannot really use a kinaesthetic system: you cannot feel a word to spell it correctly. Sometimes you can write a word and just have a feeling that it is not right, but that does not help you to actually spell it correctly. Therefore, perhaps a different strategy is worth trying:

- Write down the capital of Iceland.

- Compare your version with the correct spelling. If you got it right, then well done. If you didn't, do not be discouraged; you will probably never need to spell it anyway! The problem with the word is that there are too many digits. We tend to struggle with words or telephone numbers that contain more than seven digits, unless they are our own number or a number that we use constantly.

- Try to spell it visually. Write down the first part of the word. Then, when it is written on your paper, hold the paper up so that you have to look up to your left to see it (to the right if you are left-handed). Then see it up there, close your eyes and visualise it. Once you have done that, put the paper down and write the second part of the word. Hold it up to the left and go through the same process of closing your eyes and seeing it with your eyes closed (but do not do this in the exam, by the way). Once you have done that, write the last part down and follow the same process. If you have done it correctly when you come to spell the word, you will use visual memory and look up to the left to retrieve the word.

The key point of this exercise is simply this – if your strategy does not work in helping you to remember what you need to for the exam, try something else.

Being in the Exam

The other issue to address is actually being in the examination room with invigilators or assessors watching over you. If you do get anxious in exams, try these top tips:

- Try to relax your muscles. When we feel anxious we tend to tense up (like you do when you're in the dentist's chair). When muscles tense up, the process spreads. Your legs start to tense up when there is no need for it because the chair supports you. Feeling tense can make our minds go blank. Take slow, deep breaths and try to calm your mind down. Look out of the window for a while and do not try to force your mind when it is not really ready. If you feel anxious and all you can see is a blank sheet of paper staring back up at you, then start by rewriting the question as part of your introduction. Often when we put things into our own words we tend to understand them better.

- Once you get the paper, just take a pause. Do not try to rush it. Too many candidates lose marks because as soon as they get the paper they read a question and they're off. They may not even read the question again. You probably know how easy it is to drift away from the actual question in an essay.

- Read the instructions carefully. By looking at past papers you may get an idea about the format, but usually you have a few minutes to do this in the exam. In the past, I have asked a multiple-choice question with four possible answers, 'a', 'b', 'c' or 'd'. I am always surprised when someone puts 'e' as their answer!

- If you have a choice of questions, then tick the ones you feel reasonably confident about and put a pencil line through those you don't. If you find you have a line through every question, rub the lines out and start again.

- We all have topics that we feel confident with but do not try to twist the question/scenario to one you wish you had been asked. You can only get good marks if you answer the question set. You can get higher marks by showing a depth of understanding which is often demonstrated by how your answer relates to other topics, but make sure you are answering the question set.

- Answer the easiest question or section first. That way, at least you can start banking marks. Do not spend most of the exam on the hardest question because you want to get it out of the way. You need to spend most of your time on questions you feel most confident about.

- If you wished you had answered another question instead, do not put a line through your work. Anything with a line through does not get read. You are often better off sticking to the question you have started. Leave some space and come back to it later. Very often when you start on another question you have thoughts of what you could include in your original question, as the content for one answer is very often related to another.

- Leave time at the end to re-read your work. I know you do not like doing this but in an exam you tend to write quicker and you can miss little words out. For example, 'Rogers was a behaviourist theorist' instead of 'Rogers was *not* a behaviourist theorist'. The marker cannot make an assumption as to what they think you meant.

- If you are short of time, get the main points down. The marker may well see that you do know your stuff and could give you credit for it.

- If you have multiple-choice questions, try to answer the question yourself first before you look at the answers. Do not put two answers in the hope that you think you have got a 50:50 chance of getting a mark. Also, make sure that you at least attempt each question even if it is a guess.

One final point – do not leave early thinking that it's cool to be the first one to do so. Those who leave early tend to be the ones who do not do well.

Good luck!

Reference

O'Connor, J. and Seymour, J. (1990) *Introducing NLP: Psychological Skills for Understanding and Influencing People*, HarperElement, London.

Index

Locators in **bold** refer to tables

Rapid Midwifery, First Edition. Sarah Snow, Kate Taylor, and Jane Carpenter.
© 2016 John Wiley & Sons, Ltd. Published 2016 by John Wiley & Sons, Ltd.